Dr. Curtis's Guide To Staying Healthy with Science Based Non-Pharmacological Medicine

Dr. C.M. Curtis DC BCCT FIACT
Dr. C.M. Curtis

Contents

Introduction

No one wants to die young, but being old and sick is not a lot of fun, either.

Degenerative diseases, including type 2 diabetes, cancer, heart disease, autoimmune disease, and others, are running rampant in modern society, and the true causes are not being addressed.

The purpose of this book is to provide heavily researched, scientific information to people who want to live a long and HEALTHY life and are searching for fresh knowledge (and, in some cases, ancient illumination) to guide them.

Long before the internet and before functional medicine was a thing, Dr. Curtis began researching and studying science-based, natural methods of lifestyle and healing to better enable people to get well, stay well, and enjoy a long and healthy life.

For over 40 years, in addition to his clinical work, Dr. Curtis has shared his extensive knowledge as a health and nutrition advocate by serving as a talk radio host, newspaper columnist, college professor, writer, and public speaker.

Today, he pursues his passion for teaching about alternative modes of health and healing through videos he creates and shares on his social media platforms.

Chapter One

Is Alternative Medicine Science-Based?

What is Science-Based Medicine?

We often hear or read the term "science-based medicine." And it seems to always be in the context of 'as opposed to natural medicine.' In other words, drugs and surgery are science-based. Natural healing agents are not.

The thinking behind this is very simple. It's also about as far from being scientific as it could get.

If we're going to believe in and follow science—and we should—then let's do it. Let's not just pretend. And, in order to act in a truly scientific way, we have to think in a truly scientific way. We have to follow all the rules of scientific philosophy. But, it's been my observation that the people who scream "science, science, science" the loudest are almost always the ones who break most of the important rules of scientific thinking and behavior.

What they are really saying, without realizing it is, "Don't use your own brain, don't follow the rules of true scientific reasoning, just think the way I want you to think—because I'm just thinking the way someone else tells me to think, and you are wrong if you don't do the same.

Here are some of the most important scientific rules that are also some of the most often broken and ignored.

Approach every issue with open-minded skepticism. In other words, do not blindly reject or accept anything without doing your own research and analyzing the issue objectively from all possible viewpoints.

Do not begin any form of research or experiment, formal or informal, with an end result in mind. Seek only to learn the truth, whatever it may be.

Do not make the mistake of believing everything you are told/taught by people who are experts or authorities in their field. No matter how much they know, they will always be wrong or misinformed about some things.

Remember; that which we call science is constantly changing. Every generation of doctors and scientists looks back on past generations of doctors and scientists with ridicule and disdain for the now-disproven things they believed and practiced. But every new generation believes that what they are taught and what their generation believes is all true, not realizing that future generations will look back on them too, with ridicule and disdain.

Be humble. Be teachable. To be otherwise is unscientific.

Always remember that, with the exception of the latest drug, new advances in medicine and science are never new. They are usually at least 20 to 50 years old, and the originators may be dead and were probably ridiculed and persecuted—in some cases even assassinated—simply because they were ahead of their time and they threatened the status quo.

Never forget that in any major realm of human endeavor, at any given time, there is always a mainstream, and the mainstream is always right about some things and always wrong about others. The things the mainstream is right about tend to make mainstream thinkers believe they are right about everything. Mainstream thinkers are the sheep of the world. They always stick with the majority, only believing the things they believe because almost everyone else believes them.

Very few mainstreamers (if they even thought about it) would admit, even to themselves, that they are mainstream thinkers.

Mainstream thinking is safe and comfortable. Thinking outside the mainstream is uncomfortable and brings on persecution from mainstreamers, who hate nonconformists.

Don't be a nonconformist just for the sake of nonconformity. People who do that are merely mainstreamers putting on a show. Only seek knowledge and truth. They will come at a cost, but they are worth it.

Having said all that, let's analyze the concept of 'science-based' as it relates to the mainstream healthcare field.

As previously stated, people who use the term 'science-based medicine' are usually referring to allopathic (conventional) medicine (in other words; drugs and surgery) as opposed to natural medicine, holistic medicine, alternative medicine, functional medicine, or whatever you choose to call it. Those people are mainstreamers, and their minds will not open up to the possibility that the natural realm of healing could be science-based.

But is it?

Is natural medicine really science-based?

One of many places where the answer to that question can be found is PubMed, the website of the National Institutes of Health. PubMed is where everyone who is anyone in the field of health research publishes the results of their research. There are over 37 million studies reported on PubMed and it is growing daily.

Many of those studies report on natural substances i.e. herbs, amino acids, vitamins, minerals, etc. And, in many cases, the results prove specific health benefits bestowed by the natural substance(s) being studied.

I could give many examples, and I have done so in other articles, but let it be understood that natural healing as it is practiced today is based on mountains of valid scientific research.

Much of the research conducted on natural substances, particularly on herbs, is and has been funded by pharmaceutical companies, with the aim of discovering what compound(s) are present in specific herbs that give the herbs their healing properties. The goal is to Isolate the active compound(s) of a beneficial herb and then find a way to synthesize that compound and create a new drug.

In other words, the pharmaceutical industry believes in herbs.

Of course, they do.

Consider this statement from article PMC9579558 on PubMed:

"Plants are a source of a wide range of natural products that possess various therapeutic properties and are continuously explored to develop novel drugs. For ages, traditional medicines have depended on these natural products to treat many diseases. Today, most of the pharmaceutical medications are processed from these natural products."

In the natural realm of healing, we use the scientifically established therapeutic properties of healing herbs and other natural substances to bring about health and longevity, in most cases without harmful side effects.

We work with nature, not against it.

Chapter Two

GERD – Think You Have Excess Stomach Acid? Maybe the Reverse is True

Proper function of the digestive system is essential for good health. If you suffer from GERD (gastroesophageal reflux disease), your digestive system is not functioning properly, and a host of other health problems may result. If you are like me, and acid-reducing drugs are something you definitely do not want in your body, you're in luck. Get ready for a science lesson—the science of human digestion, to be precise. And when you're finished, I guarantee you'll have a whole new perspective on the subject of gastroesophageal reflux disease, otherwise known as GERD, heartburn, excess stomach acid, indigestion, hyperacidity and a few other, mostly erroneous, names.

Excess stomach acid is a common misdiagnosis

Why erroneous? Because most of the time, the diagnosis and treatment of GERD are based on the false concept that, for some unknown reason, the stomach is producing too much acid. And it really is a false concept. I'll explain why in a minute, but first, keeping in mind that GERD is much more common in people over the age of 45, let me ask a question. As we age, how many of our physical functions increase? Do we have more energy? Does our eyesight improve? Do we have better skin or more hair? Do our muscles get stronger? Do sexual desire and function increase? Does our elimination improve?

I could go on, but you get the message. It's no secret that as our age goes up, our physical functions go down. But when it comes to our digestion, we are expected to believe that many of us produce more stomach acid than we used to. Too much, in fact. It's simply not true. In reality, most people over the age of forty produce substantially less hydrochloric acid than they did when they were younger. How do you know if you are in that group? Well, one very good indicator is that you have the symptoms that are commonly diagnosed as being related to excess acid. Stay with me as I explain the physiology behind this seeming paradox.

Here's how your digestive process works

Here's how it works: There is a valve at either end of the stomach; the lower esophageal sphincter (L.E.S.) at the top (this is the one-way valve that allows food and fluids to flow from the esophagus into the stomach) and the pyloric valve at the bottom (this is the valve that releases the digested contents of the stomach into the first part of the small intestine). The pyloric valve will not open to allow the stomach contents out until they are sufficiently alkaline, and this alkalinity is not supposed to occur until proper and complete digestion has taken place. But, because you are deficient in acid, your last meal just sits there, digesting far too slowly. Your stomach is churning the food as it's supposed to do, but digestion is taking too long, and as a result, the stomach wall becomes inflamed (often chronically), and the valve at the top of the stomach weakens and leaks stomach contents into the esophagus, causing the burning sensation known as GERD, or heartburn. So, you reach for an antacid. When you do this, you further reduce the acidity of the stomach, temporarily alleviating the burning sensation but setting yourself up for some serious, long-term problems.

Acid-reducing drugs have a lot of side effects

Those side effects include osteoporosis, colitis, SIBO, H-pylori, increased risk of kidney, liver, cardiovascular disease, dementia, and malabsorption of nutrients (a very bad thing), to name just a few.

WARNING: Any medication that reduces the amount of acid in your stomach is harmful to your health. These medications are based on the false premise that the problem is caused by too much acid. The best approach to this problem is to increase the amount of acid in the stomach and provide for normal, speedy, comfortable digestion. And guess what? It works.

Here are a few suggestions:

Kick the junk food out of your life! You know you need to do it for your health and longevity anyway, so why not now? Eliminate the sugar, caffeine, artificial sweeteners, inflammatory oils, gluten, etc. Also, you should eliminate any foods to which you are sensitive.

Don't drink fluids with meals. Let your digestive juices do their work without being diluted. An exception to this rule would be to drink a teaspoonful of apple cider vinegar in ½ cup of warm water just before each meal.

Take a good trace mineral supplement. These need to be ionic minerals. The ones I recommend are from seawater or the water of the Great Salt Lake

Eat plenty of fresh, raw, organic fruits and vegetables.

Eat some ginger root and a little cayenne (if your stomach tolerates it) each day.

GERD is one of those health conditions in which a simple visit to your local health food store (or online) can often make all the difference in terms of assisting the body in correcting the causes of hypochlorhydria (insufficient stomach acid).

A simple natural supplement, betaine HCL with pepsin, preferably accompanied by digestive enzymes (another thing we produce less of as we age), usually works well without the very nasty side effects of antacids and other medications—such as proton pump inhibitors (PPIs)—that reduce the amount of acid in the stomach.

It works the same way your natural stomach acid does

Betaine HCL works the same as hydrochloric acid in your stomach, so you'll need to learn to adjust the amount you take according to how well it works and how much protein you have eaten. You can take too much, but if you do, ½ to 1 tsp of baking soda in a glass of water will immediately neutralize it.

A quick-relief hack for heartburn

And, speaking of baking soda, if you ever need quick relief from heartburn/GERD, baking soda in water is a very effective and fast first aid remedy, and it doesn't carry with it the side effects of medical acid reducers and antacids.

Chapter Three

News Flash: Bone Health Is Not About Calcium

Disclaimer: I have invested many hours of research into the writing of this report. Much of the information it contains is controversial, and much of it does not align with the preponderance of information on this subject that a superficial internet search would yield. But isn't that always the case? All I can guarantee is that I have made every effort to sort out the valid science from the junk or outdated science and I personally am convinced of the validity of the information provided herein. Moreover, in view of the fact that the things I recommend avoiding for purposes of bone health are all harmful to the body in other ways and the things I recommend to protect and improve bone health are beneficial to human health in many other ways, I'm confident that anyone who follows these recommendations will benefit.

A Parable

As an introduction to this topic, I offer a parable, which I have named The Parable of The Shallow-Thinking Mechanic.

Once upon a time, there was a man who owned a car. The car was not new, and one day, the man observed some rust spots on its chassis and frame. Concerned, he took the car to a mechanic, who did a thorough examination and said, "This car has a deficiency of metal." He explained that the car's basic structure was composed of metal, and it was obvious that some of the metal had been lost.

This seemed logical to the car owner, and he trusted the mechanic. He said, "What can I do?"

"You have to add metal to the car," replied the mechanic, and he explained how this was to be done.

So, the man, following the mechanic's instructions, began adding metal to the car. He purchased a quantity of steel bars and ball bearings, and each day, he faithfully put some of them in the back seat, the trunk, the hood compartment, and even the front passenger's seat.

At first, things seemed to be going well, but with time, the accumulation of metal in the car began to cause problems with the car's functioning and operation. Moreover, the rusting away of the structure of the car continued unabated because the issue had not been truly addressed. Eventually, the combination of the weight of the "supplemental metal" and the lack of dealing with the car's real needs resulted in the car breaking down, falling apart, and having to be scrapped.

In osteoporosis, the bone matrix breaks down, and there are different factors that can cause this breakdown. It is my opinion that most people in Western society do not have calcium deficiency. In the above parable it wasn't a deficiency of metal that was causing the deterioration of the car, and adding metal only created more problems. Likewise, in osteoporosis, adding calcium to the body will no more rectify the problem than adding metal to the car stopped its deterioration. In fact, it will cause more problems, serious ones.

Much Ado Over Calcium

Much ado is made over calcium in our society while we ignore the fact that most people are seriously deficient in many, if not most, of the other important components, including minerals and certain vitamins that are also essential to bone health. These elements are necessary for the proper function of every organ, system, and cell in the body, and they are largely neglected in modern society. It is short-sighted to neglect the body's crying need for these essential elements while adding large amounts of calcium, which the body simply can't handle.

I am well aware that your doctor, your favorite health magazine, your nutritionist, the internet, and society, in general, have pounded into your consciousness the fact that calcium supplementation will preserve bone density and protect against fractures of the hip and other bones but increasing numbers of researchers are refuting that claim.

Bones are not made of just calcium, as we have all been led to believe, but of collagen (which is the main constituent of bone), 11 other minerals in significant amounts, and trace amounts of many others.

Too Much of a Good Thing Can Kill You

While it's true that calcium is an essential mineral in the body and that if a person is deficient in it, they should eat more calcium-rich foods, too many people have too much of it in their bodies already. Their cells are overloaded with calcium, which is a serious problem. According to Robert Thompson M.D., and Kathleen Barnes, two researchers on this subject, adding more calcium to an already over-loaded cell results in what is called The Calcium Cascade. This begins with excess dietary calcium and results in the following:

Suppression of the adrenal glands

Urinary loss of potassium and sodium creates health-threatening deficiencies.

Deficient production of crucially important stomach acid.

Improper digestion and assimilation of proteins.

Dangerous deficiencies in amino acids and poor cellular absorption thereof.

Calcium excess can also result in calcium being deposited in areas where it doesn't belong, areas of soft tissue where the hardening and stiffening effects of calcium are not desirable, such as muscles, joints, blood vessels, internal organs, glands, eyes, anywhere but bones and teeth where it belongs.

Calcium Supplements Can Cause Disease

Over time, calcium excess and the resulting calcium cascade can cause disease and even death. The abnormal deposition of calcium into the wrong places can also cause disease and death. Researchers in Australia reported that, in women taking calcium supplements, they observed a 17% increase in kidney stones, a 100% increase in hospital admissions for gastrointestinal side effects, and a 20–40% increase in heart attacks. (Remember, 50% of heart attacks are fatal). Other studies, including one published in the Journal of the American Heart Association, also showed an association between calcium supplements and increased risk of cardiovascular disease. Still, another study showed that calcium supplements may cause intestinal polyps, which can turn cancerous. Further studies have shown a potential correlation between calcium supplementation and strokes.

The Best Calcium Supplement is None

Johns Hopkins University seems to be on the cutting edge of this issue. In an article in johnshopkinsmedicine.org the following statement appears: The best calcium supplement is none.

More Hazards of Calcium Supplementation

In the Johns Hopkins article referenced above, Dr. Erin Michos, MD, MHS, makes the following statements: "A nutrient in pill form is not processed in the body the same way as it is when ingested from a food source. Furthermore, people believe that the proof that calcium supplements fortify bones is more robust than it really is," she says. "The truth is the research is inconclusive. But there is a growing body of evidence that suggests no health benefit, or even worse, that calcium supplements may be harmful." "I'm very concerned about the potential for calcium supplements to contribute to heart attacks and heart disease," says Michos. "The body can't process more than 500 milligrams of calcium at a time. If you take a supplement with more than that, your body has to do something with the excess. It's possible that higher calcium levels in the blood could trigger blood clots or that calcium could be deposited along artery walls, which would contribute to the narrowing of blood vessels."

It appears that the recommended daily allowances are harming people

According to Dr. Michos, the body can't process more than 500 milligrams of calcium at a time, yet the standard recommendation for post-menopausal women is 1200 milligrams per day. For men, it's 1,000 milligrams per day. Many people take their recommended daily dose in supplement form and then get a lot more calcium from their diet. This is alarming.

What About Dairy?

When the subject of calcium-rich foods is raised, most people think immediately of dairy products. But to my way of thinking, that's too broad a category. I would divide dairy into two general categories:

Commercial milk, yogurt, cheese etc, that have been pasteurized, homogenized, standardized, and very much altered from the substance that came out of the cow, and contain harmful amounts of pesticides (glyphosate being just one of them), antibiotics, synthetic hormones (in many cases), chemicals from fertilizers, and miscellaneous other chemicals.

Organic, raw grass-fed dairy products which contain none of the above but do contain beneficial substances (like CLA) and have not been significantly altered from the natural product that nature created.

Bet you can't guess which one I prefer.

The Nurses' Health Study, conducted by researchers at Harvard and Cornell Universities, one of the largest investigations ever into the risk factors for major diseases in women, shed a whole new light on dairy products for bone health. The study showed that the women who had the highest consumption of calcium from dairy products (commercial dairy products, no doubt) had substantially more fractures than women who consumed less dairy. Hmm.

Of the foods that have a negative impact on bone health, sugar tops the list. Others are caffeine, soda pop, soy (fermented soy products are OK), and junk food in general. These things have been shown to cause bone demineralization. Soda pop, in addition to containing sugar and, in most cases, caffeine, contains phosphoric acid, another offender.

Alcohol and tobacco are two more culprits. Yes, in addition to all the other ways in which these two killers harm the body, they can cause bone demineralization.

What about salt?

Well, it appears we have blamed the wrong crystal.

For years women have been cautioned to decrease their salt intake on the basis that it causes mineral loss in bones, yet, nothing was said about sugar. In a study published in Missouri Medicine in 2018, the following statement was made: In summary, it appears we have blamed the wrong crystal: it's not salt, but sugar that presents the greater risk factor for osteoporosis.

So, we can now add osteoporosis to the very long list of diseases caused by sugar.

Here are some things that can truly improve bone health and prevent osteoporosis

In addition to calcium, many healthcare professionals recommend vitamin D3 for its numerous health benefits, including bone health. The problem with this recommendation is that vitamin D only helps with bone density when it is accompanied by vitamin K2.* In fact, vitamin D can actually be harmful if there are insufficient levels of vitamin K2 in the body. And, an estimated 80 to 85 percent of people in Western society are deficient in K2. K2 is also beneficial to heart and brain function, and it activates many of the benefits of vitamin D3.

It is important to maintain the correct ratio of K2 to D3; therefore, people who take higher amounts of D3 need to get more K2 in their bodies as well. According to current scientific literature, a good ratio is 100-200 mcg of K2 for every 1,000 IU of D3 taken. You don't have to worry about taking too much K2. This vitamin, unlike other fat-soluble vitamins, has no known toxic level. There is no down-side to ingesting high amounts of K2 (also known as K2,7, MK7, or Menaquinone)

Vitamin K2 protects against degenerative diseases

In addition to osteoporosis, a deficiency of vitamin K2 results in a greater risk of heart disease, cancer, kidney stones, neurodegenerative diseases (like Alzheimer's), and other undesirable diseases.

The point is that, in view of the fact that there is a crying need in our bodies for vitamin D3, vitamin K2, and more than 75 trace minerals, supplementation of just one mineral (almost always calcium) is just plain silly. Furthermore, as I have pointed out, it could be dangerous.

Here's what you can do to protect your bone health

First of all, you should avoid the things on the list of offenders above.

Then, get plenty of sunlight and exercise. Eat foods that are high in K2, like grass-fed foods, fermented vegetables, butter (especially grass-fed), egg yolks (organic), certain cheeses (like gouda and brie), goose pate and natto (natto is super high in K2).

Get plenty of good sleep. Chronic sleep deprivation has been shown to contribute to osteoporosis.

Here is a list of nutrients I recommend for their positive effect on bone health and mineralization. (Some of them are mentioned above.)

Vitamin K2, 7 (MK7)

Vitamin D3 (Remember, vitamin D can actually be harmful unless you are getting sufficient amounts of Vitamin K2)

Camu Camu powder (for its extremely high content of vitamin C and numerous other health-promoting elements)

Magnesium Glycinate (All magnesium supplements are not created equal).

- Lutein

- Boron

- Strontium

- Zinc picolinate

- Tocotrienols

- Collagen

Ionic trace minerals (preferably from the sea or the Great Salt Lake. And be sure they are ionic).

Beneficial foods

Please don't think I'm an enemy of calcium. We need it for life. It's best, however, to get it from foods, and, as previously stated, too much is a bad thing. If you are concerned that you may be deficient in the mineral, here are some foods that are high in calcium.

Dried figs

Broccoli

Dark green leafy vegetables such as kale, spinach, collard greens, and Bok choy.

Garbanzos, white beans, black beans, and pinto beans.

I have given my thoughts on dairy products above.

*Vitamin K is often confused with potassium due to the fact that the chemical symbol for potassium is K. But potassium is a mineral, and vitamin K is – obviously – a vitamin.

Chapter Four

Cholesterophobia– Do you have it?

Two historical figures that fascinate me are Will Rogers and Albert Einstein. My interest in them has to do with the fact that they both said so many profoundly wise things, many of them couched in humor. One of my favorite Will Rogers quotes is: "It ain't what we don't know that gives us trouble; it's what we know that ain't so." Homespun, though it may sound, this is a profound piece of wisdom, and it is from this vantage point that I propose we begin our look at the cholesterol issue. Let's start with a list of what we think we know:

What we think we know:

Cholesterol is bad, and it causes cardiovascular disease.

Cholesterol-lowering drugs protect against cardiovascular disease.

Eggs and other foods that are high in cholesterol raise blood cholesterol and should be avoided.

In recent decades, cholesterol has been demonized to such an extent that most people suffer from what is known as cholesterophobia. In the clinical setting, I couldn't count the times patients came to me for blood tests, wanting to know if they 'had cholesterol,' as if it were some sort of disease. And, indeed, so it has been portrayed.

Allow me – lest the universe become unbalanced and topple on its side – to give the other side of the story and cast cholesterol in its rightful role as the hero: Simply put, without cholesterol, life would be impossible. It is the primary component of our cell membranes, not to mention the stuff from which vitamin D and steroid hormones (estrogens, progesterone, testosterone, etc.) are made. Furthermore, your liver produces most of the cholesterol that is circulating in your bloodstream at any given time.

Why would it do that? Why would your liver produce something that is going to cause you to have a heart attack or a stroke? The best answer to that question is that it doesn't. We have solid science that shows that cholesterol is not a major player in the rampant plague of heart disease that only in the last hundred years, and mostly in the last fifty years, has afflicted our society.

A 2018 article published in Expert Review of Clinical Pharmacology bore the following title:

LDL-C does not cause cardiovascular disease. (LDL-C stands for LDL-cholesterol or low-density lipoprotein cholesterol)

Put in lay terms, the primary conclusion of the article, which was a review of 107 published scientific studies, was that LDL cholesterol, which has been blamed for decades as being the cause of atherosclerosis (arterial plaquing), is not guilty.

The article cites multiple studies that show there is no connection between cholesterol and cardiovascular disease. Many people who have heart attacks and strokes have low cholesterol levels, and there are many people whose cholesterol levels are higher than the 'recommended levels' who never suffer any cardiovascular disease.

In fact, the authors of the article make the following extraordinary statement:

Elderly people with high LDL-C (LDL Cholesterol) live the longest.

The authors go on to say:

If high LDL-C was the major cause of atherosclerosis and CVD, people with the highest LDL-C should have shorter lives than people with low values. However, in a recent systematic review of 19 cohort studies including more than 68,000 elderly people (>60 years of age), we found the opposite: those with the highest LDL-C levels lived even longer than those on statin treatment. In addition, numerous Japanese studies have found that high LDL-C is not a risk factor for CHD (congestive heart disease) mortality in women of any age.

The authors of the article also make the following statement:

The association between TC (total cholesterol) and CVD (cardiovascular disease) is weak, absent, or inverse in many studies.

So, as I see it, this brings into focus two huge problems. The first is that cardiovascular disease, which has risen from a rare disease to being the number one cause of death in our society, continues to rise, and the true causes are not being addressed. The second is that tens of millions of people are taking Statin drugs to lower their cholesterol and are being exposed to the very serious side effects of those drugs.

Cholesterol, if it needs to be lowered at all, can be lowered using scientific, natural alternative methods, without the risks and side effects of Statin drugs.

There are hundreds of studies proving the hazards of taking Statin drugs. These include type 2 diabetes, inflammation of the liver and pancreas, hair loss, abdominal issues, skin rash, acne, neuropathy, depression, and muscle problems ranging from weakness to severe degeneration (this affects the heart as well – it is, after all, a muscle), cataracts, sexual dysfunction (including erectile dysfunction), pancreas and liver dysfunction, anemia, acidosis (a potentially fatal condition), cognitive impairment (including poor memory, difficulty concentrating, even disorientation) and a lot more.

Quite often, people who are experiencing side effects of statin drugs are told that their symptoms are due to their age, and if you look at the list, you will recognize a number of the potential side effects as being common symptoms of aging. These people are generally prescribed other drugs to deal with the statin side effects. There have been many cases in which individuals were diagnosed with Alzheimer's disease because of cognitive changes and disorientation, but when the Statin drugs were discontinued, the symptoms disappeared.

Here, we have a situation in which billions of dollars are spent annually to treat the symptoms of a problem as we watch the incidence of that problem continue to rise unabated, yet we do nothing about true prevention.

Albert Einstein said: "No problem can be solved from the same level of consciousness that created it." What has created this horrific situation that is our number one cause of death and each year claims more lives than the last? The answer couldn't possibly be more obvious: Our unnatural lifestyle, our unnatural foods, and our unnatural environment. And how are we addressing the situation? With something that is more unnatural than the original causes of the problem.

Eggs don't raise blood cholesterol

As a side note on the subject of prevention, avoiding eggs is not helpful. In fact, dietary cholesterol is not a significant factor in elevated serum cholesterol. Tests have failed to demonstrate any significant change in blood cholesterol levels when test subjects consumed large numbers of eggs daily for months. I'm not saying that dietary factors don't play a major role in elevated cholesterol; they most certainly do, but you may be surprised to learn that sugar, seed oils, trans fats, and deficiencies of Vitamin C and certain B vitamins are much more the culprits than are eggs or most types of fats in the cardiovascular disease scenario. In fact, eating the right fats is an extremely important aspect of good cardiovascular health.

One of the most routinely performed blood tests is the total cholesterol test, which is, unfortunately, a very poor indicator of cardiovascular disease risk. Far better tests are homocysteine and CRP – both very strong indicators of risk – and the HDL/Total Cholesterol Ratio, which, unlike total cholesterol alone, can be a useful test.

If you take Statin drugs, I strongly recommend that you take a quality, high potency Coenzyme Q10 supplement daily as well as a healthy amount of vitamin K2 (MK7) either from foods or in supplement form to protect your body from some of the effects of the drug.

There are natural substances that work very well in controlling serum cholesterol levels, with additional health benefits as well.

I believe we can cut through the cholesterol/statin controversy very easily by simply discussing a number of natural things that have been researched scientifically and shown to normalize blood cholesterol. In view of the fact that statin drugs have only one purpose – to lower cholesterol levels – if you are able to normalize your cholesterol levels without them, your doctor will surely not prescribe a statin. And everyone will be happy. You'll be happy to be able to avoid the side effects of statins, your doctor will be happy not to have to write another prescription, and your body will be happy to have all the additional health benefits of the natural medicines listed below. It will be a winning situation all the way around – whether you believe in the cholesterol theory or not.

Cue the happy dance. Here's the list. (these have all been proven in scientific studies to lower cholesterol)

Bergamot: This amazing natural medicine has many additional benefits, like blood sugar control, elevating HDL (so-called good cholesterol), and others.

Berberine: Like bergamot, this one can also lower blood sugar levels along with numerous other health benefits.

Vitamin K2: I couldn't list all the benefits this important vitamin offers.

Gugulipid: Also good for the thyroid, acne, inflammation, lowering triglycerides, and as an antioxidant.

Camu Powder: Another one with countless health benefits.

Vitamin B6, B12 and folate

Krill oil: (fish oil also works, but krill is a better source of omega-3 fatty acids). Also provides multiple health benefits.

Garlic: It goes without saying garlic offers tons of benefits to the body.

Magnesium: (I recommend magnesium taurate for this purpose). The master mineral. Over 600 functions that we know of in the body.

Olive oil: Another one with multiple benefits.

There are others, as well. All of these natural medicines are easily found in health food stores and online.

I just say no to red yeast rice

As a side note, I don't recommend red yeast rice, because of the chemicals it contains and because of the precautions and side effects associated with it. There are so many natural medicines that are effective in controlling serum cholesterol without significant side effects, that I fail to see the need for red yeast rice.

Inflammation causes atherosclerosis

Inflammation of the arterial wall causes arterial plaquing (atherosclerosis). There are multiple causes of this inflammation. Vitamin C deficiency is one of them, and for this, I recommend Camu powder.

Camu is a fruit from the South American rainforest, and it contains the highest vitamin C content of any food we know of, 30 to 60 times as much as an orange, and it is natural vitamin C, accompanied by all the cofactors that assist in assimilation of the vitamin. I prefer it over any other source of vitamin C, especially supplements, which tend to be poorly assimilated, even, in some cases, causing the body to lose vitamin C.

Another cause of arterial wall inflammation is homocysteine, an amino acid produced when certain proteins are broken down. High homocysteine can contribute to arterial wall damage and blood clots. However, if there are sufficient amounts of vitamin B6, B12, and folate in the body, the homocysteine is broken down into cysteine and methionine, which are beneficial and do not cause inflammation or arterial wall damage.

Chapter Five

UTIs, Bladder Infections, and the 90% Miracle

I often speak and write about the scientific nature of today's alternative medicine, and there is a treatment for urinary tract infections that is a perfect example of that concept. I frequently tell my patients and readers that I am a big fan of conventional medicine, and I truly am. Just like I'm a fan of each tool in my toolbox. But no matter how much I like a particular tool, I will only use it for the job for which it is designed and only when it is the best choice for the job. Just because I don't recommend using a saw to drive nails doesn't mean I don't believe in saws or don't reach for one when I need to cut a board.

I approach health care in the same way. When I feel that a patient needs conventional medicine, I recommend it. But if there is a viable, natural alternative to drugs or surgery, I will choose the natural alternative every time.

Women get UTIs (urinary tract infections) more often than men. Some women (and men) never get them, others get them occasionally, and for other women, the problem is a constant nightmare. The standard medical treatment for the condition is antibiotic therapy.

Antibiotics are a double-edged sword

Everyone knows that antibiotics are a double-edged sword. I'm glad we have them. They sometimes save lives, but they have their downside, too. They have side effects, which in some cases are worse than the disease they are being used to treat. Antibiotics don't know when to stop killing. They don't know good bacteria from bad bacteria. They just kill. One of the common side effects of antibiotics is the destruction of the beneficial bacteria in the body. They are referred to as beneficial bacteria, but I call them essential bacteria because they are essential to good health, and when they are killed, serious health problems are unavoidable. And, these health problems are seldom recognized as having been caused by the patient's previous antibiotic use.

Super-infections are a huge and growing menace to our health

Another very dangerous consequence of antibiotic therapy is the creation of the so-called superbugs. These are the bacteria that have become immune or resistant to antibiotics and are extremely difficult—in some cases even impossible to kill. Every day many people die from these deadly infections. Two of the more common and well-known of the superbugs are MRSA (Methicillin-resistant Staphylococcus Aureus) and C-Diff (Clostridium difficile).

Fungal overgrowth—another hazard of antibiotics

Another of the many side effects of antibiotic therapy is fungal overgrowth, usually a common fungus known as candida albicans. This fungus can cause devastation in the health of the individual who has an overgrowth of it (candidiasis), and in most cases, it goes untreated—even undiagnosed, while the patient's doctor treats only the symptoms that arise from the huge quantities of toxins produced by this pernicious fungus.

Most women know that the right antibiotic will usually kill a UTI. They also know that quite often, soon after the UTI is gone, they will get a vaginal yeast (fungal) infection.

Why?

Destruction of the protective bacteria leaves the body vulnerable to fungal infection

It's very simple. The beneficial bacteria in the vagina (the vaginal flora), are protective. One of their functions is to prevent the overgrowth of dangerous organisms like Candida Albicans (yeast). When the vaginal flora is killed by the antibiotic, the fungus takes over, and the problems begin. Of course, there are medications to kill the fungus, but without flora replacement, they do not correct the causes of the problem, which is why so many women suffer from chronic vaginitis and/or recurrent yeast infections. This can affect the bladder, resulting in the well-known infection-antibiotic-infection cycle. (A similar cycle often occurs when ear infections are treated with antibiotic therapy, but that's a subject for another article).

Yeast infection is fungal (typically candida albicans)

To make matters worse, when a woman gets a yeast infection it's pretty much a sure bet, she has the candida fungus in the intestinal tract. From there, it usually goes throughout the body and the person (men get candida too) now has systemic candidiasis—a condition that many doctors refuse to diagnose or even accept, and which conventional medicine has very few tools to deal with effectively or safely.

Fortunately, in the natural realm of healing, we have effective treatments for individuals who suffer from candidiasis. And the problem is more common than you may know. I have done videos on candida, and I will do an article on it soon.

We come back to the concept of using less damaging alternatives when they are available. And, in the case of urinary tract infections, there's something that fits the bill perfectly.

D-Mannose, a safe, effective, scientific natural alternative

It's called D-mannose.

D-Mannose is a natural sugar, but don't think of it as sugar because, other than the fact that it's sweet, it does not do to you the things that common table sugar does, like make you gain weight or cause diabetes, etc. Nor is D-Mannose an antibiotic, natural or otherwise, so there are none of the standard antibiotic side effects.

How effective is D-Mannose? Very effective. In fact, published studies have shown it to be as effective as antibiotics. And side effects are rare and mild, consisting only of loose stools. Better yet, D-Mannose can be purchased online or in almost any health food store. It only works on urinary tract infections that are caused by E. coli, but, according to the National Kidney Foundation, up to 90 percent of UTIs are caused by E-coli so the odds are in your favor. In many years of practice, I have rarely seen D-Mannose fail.

And, for people who suffer from chronic recurring infections D-Mannose taken correctively will usually stop the infection, and, used preventively it can end the destructive cycle. Yes, because D-Mannose is so safe, you can take it daily (I recommend it at bedtime) to prevent ever having another UTI.

Children, dogs, and cats too

And, as a side note, children, dogs, and cats can take D-Mannose as well, and experience the same benefits.

There was a time when the only doctors who were prescribing D-Mannose were those who practiced natural forms of healing, but these days, because of the mountains of scientific research showing the effectiveness and safety of D-Mannose, increasing numbers of medical doctors, even urologists are prescribing it. And it has been written up in many prestigious medical journals.

Unfortunately, however, there are still far too many medical doctors who are stuck in their backward ways and continue to prescribe antibiotics for UTIs, subjecting their patients to the risks and hazards of that outdated approach.

Here's how to take D-Mannose

I have seen that the best way to take D-Mannose is in powder form, not capsules. An effective way to take the powder is one teaspoonful in a glass of water every two waking hours on the first day of use, the same dosage (1 teaspoonful) every three hours on the second day, and then every four hours on the third day, continuing at every four hours until the symptoms are resolved. After this, it is a good idea to take a teaspoonful of D-Mannose every night at bedtime for a week or two just to make sure the bacteria is completely gone. If you have a chronic problem of frequent bladder infections this bedtime maintenance dosage will usually keep the infection from recurring.

D-Mannose is healthy and safe, and the bacteria cannot develop resistance to it.

The effectiveness and safety of D-Mannose is supported by numerous studies

Below, I have cited some of the many published studies confirming the effectiveness (equal to that of antibiotics) and safety of D-Mannose in treating patients who suffer from UTIs. These studies can all be found on PubMed Central

Antibiotics Mar 11. 2022

Antibiotics Apr 1. 2021

Healthline Medical News Nov 2019

Molecules Jan 25, 2020

HHS Author manuscripts Mar 25, 2022

The list could go on and on. There are many published studies showing the effectiveness and safety of D-Mannose.

Additionally, there is ongoing research showing that D-Mannose is probably beneficial in other ways as well, such as osteoarthritis, and improving bone density.

Chapter Six

Are You Mineral Deficient? Does it really matter that much?

Does taking multivitamins with minerals really matter that much?

You take vitamins. Of course, you do

You want to do good things for your body. And you take a multivitamin with minerals in it and maybe some extra calcium on the side. That should cover it, shouldn't it?

No.

First, let's discuss the multivitamin concept

Most multivitamin products are junk. That includes the most heavily advertised national brands. Not only do those companies use the cheapest, most poorly assimilated ingredients (many of them synthetic), but the amounts of each ingredient in the pill or capsule are dismally small. I'm not saying all multivitamin products are junk, but it's simply not possible to cram everything we may need into something small enough to swallow.

And as for minerals

Formulated mineral products contain only the minerals the formulator puts in them. In most cases, you can count them on one hand, and almost always, they will include calcium—too much of it for my liking. (see my article on bone health and calcium).

It is claimed that the human body contains 102 different minerals. All but six of these are trace minerals. We don't know all the functions every trace mineral performs in our bodies, but we know many of them, and we know they are essential for life and good health, and that in many cases, vitamins, enzymes, hormones, and antioxidants are unable to perform their functions without the help of minerals. Furthermore, we know that most people are deficient in macro minerals and trace minerals.

Taking a formulated mineral supplement is not going to supply your mineral needs.

Taking a multivitamin/mineral supplement or a formulated multimineral product with a handful of minerals—in all too many cases, the wrong forms of the minerals—is not going to supply our needs.

I have written extensively about the disastrous epidemic of degenerative diseases that has only in recent times descended on our society. There are multiple factors involved in this tragedy, but for the most part, the causes can be listed under one of two headings: Things we put in our bodies that do harm, and things our bodies need that they don't get. Minerals fall under the second heading.

The science of nutritional supplementation is very complex

The science of nutritional supplementation is a complex one and it requires a solid understanding of human physiology, among other sciences. Most formulators of nutritional products seem to be lacking either in knowledge or integrity. I say this because it seems that if they had the knowledge, they would not formulate supplements with inferior ingredients. On the other hand, if they have the knowledge and they create and sell inferior products, they are clearly lacking in integrity. Either way, trusting consumers are cheated out of their money and the health benefits they hoped to derive from supplementation.

That is a long way of saying that a lot of nutritional products are garbage, and since we are talking primarily about minerals in this article, I should say that a lot of mineral supplements are garbage.

Getting a supplement into the stomach is easy; you just swallow it. Getting it into the bloodstream is not so hard either; your body can usually handle that part quite nicely. But getting it into the cells, where it has to do its work, well, that's the challenge. The only minerals that can make it into our cells are ionic minerals. So if you are going to take minerals, they should be in ionic form.

Just say no to colloidal minerals

Some years ago, there was much ado about colloidal minerals. I do not recommend them. I don't believe they can ever make it into the cell. I see them as a complete waste of money.

So, how can you know if you are trace mineral deficient?

Frankly, if you are not already taking a high-quality ionic trace mineral supplement, it's a pretty safe bet you are deficient in trace minerals. There was a time when everything humans ate was organic. And it was grown using natural fertilizers in soil that was full of nutrients and beneficial bacteria. People did not refine their salt and remove the seventy-five plus trace minerals, leaving only sodium and chloride. Furthermore, there was no fast food, soda pop, Gatorade, seed oils, or packaged, processed foods. Their water was not so contaminated that they had to filter it to remove the poisons, stripping it of its minerals in the process . . . I could go on, but you get the picture. People got their minerals from their foods, their salt, and their water. Things aren't like that anymore.

To anyone with a good understanding of human nutritional physiology, it should be abundantly clear that we need to take nutritional supplements. But we need to take the right ones.

Malnourished and overweight

I once met with a doctor from a third-world country. He made the following statement to me: "In my country, there are many skinny people who are suffering from malnutrition. Here in America, I see many obese people who are suffering from malnutrition."

Malnourished and overweight. This describes an alarming percentage of people in our modern society. When we are mineral deficient, we tend to have cravings. It's often the body's way of asking for more nutrients. However, a common tendency is to respond to this need with high glycemic foods that have very little true nutrient value.

This results in obesity coupled with malnutrition

A perfect recipe for degenerative diseases like heart disease, type 2 diabetes, and cancer—the very diseases that are running rampant in our modern society.

The solution is obvious

Eat natural salt that has not been refined. (I recommend Himalayan salt or Redmond Real Salt. I no longer recommend sea salt due to microplastic contamination of the oceans), eat natural, organic foods and take an ionic trace mineral supplement made from seawater or water from the Great Salt Lake. Most people are also deficient in potassium and magnesium, the master mineral (see my article on magnesium), so it's a good idea to supplement these two minerals as well.

Chapter Seven

Thyroid Disease – Misunderstood Epidemic

Thyroid disease, which not long ago was rare, has, in recent years, like so many other diseases, become far too common. The causes of this are manifold, having to do, to a great extent, with chemicals (many of them hormone disruptors) in our foods and in products we use and are exposed to in numerous ways. Deficiencies in certain essential nutrients, notable among them being Iodine, also contribute to the problem. This is just another example of how our modern lifestyle can destroy our health.

What about prevention?

What about it? We don't do it. We, as a society, do not seem to be able to even try to attack the roots of problems. We are not a prevention-oriented society. We throw money and political rhetoric at social problems and drugs at the symptoms of disease.

What are the causes of thyroid disease?

There are so many hormone-disrupting chemicals and thyroid-damaging foods in daily use in most people's lives that it would be difficult to list them all, but I will mention a few of the primary offenders and how to avoid them:

Non-stick coatings on cookware, etc.: Solution - Use cookware without non-stick coating.

Bromine: is found in pastry flour. Solution - Avoid these products. They cause obesity, diabetes, thyroid disease and more

Fluoride and chlorine: These are two extremely toxic chemicals, and there is research that shows they have a detrimental effect on thyroid function. Chlorine is in all municipal water supplies, and fluoride is in many of them. Solution: Avoid drinking tap water for many reasons. It's full of chemicals (more about water below), Also, there are natural toothpastes that do not contain fluoride. It's an established fact that we absorb much of the fluoride that's in our toothpaste through the highly absorbent membranes of the mouth. (children absorb more than adults.)

GMO (genetically modified) foods: These foods contain glyphosate (Roundup), a toxic herbicide that is banned in many countries (but not in the United States) due to the many diseases it causes, including cancer. Research shows it also affects the thyroid. Solution: Eating organic and non-GMO is extremely important these days.

Soy: Avoid it. It is an unhealthy substance.

Gluten: Opinions on this are mixed, but it appears that gluten may negatively impact the thyroid. Furthermore, some researchers claim that in cases of Hashimoto's thyroiditis, excluding gluten from the diet is crucial.

Freshwater fish: Heavily contaminated with PFOS (causes thyroid cancer). Solution - Avoid.

Flame retardant clothing: Avoid

Water or stain-repellent clothing or other textile products: Just say no.

Microwave popcorn: Solution: You can make your own popcorn with non-GMO popping corn and coconut oil. Put real butter on it.

Many cleaning products: Solution - Buy natural products or make your own.

Many personal care products: Solution - Buy natural products.

Fast foods: The Solution - Kick them out of your life. They are killers.

Un-purified water: Unfortunately, we have contaminated all the water on our planet, consequently drinking tap water is a very bad idea. However, drinking out of plastic bottles is also a bad idea because of chemicals and microplastics. Solution - It's best to have a reverse osmosis filter in your home (they are quite inexpensive these days) or buy water in glass bottles.

All inflammatory substances: Inflammatory substances can negatively affect the whole body, including the thyroid. The list of common inflammatory substances is too extensive to list here, but it includes substances that we already know we should avoid, like sugar, high fructose corn syrup, agave, alcohol, tobacco, monosodium glutamate, and many other poisons.

I know the above list may be a little discouraging, but actually, it's not that hard to do; I have been doing it for decades. The thing to remember is that all the thyroid-damaging offenders on the above list cause multiple other diseases, like cancer. So by avoiding them, you will give yourself a much better chance for a long and healthy life.

Deficiencies that can affect thyroid function:

One common cause of low function in the thyroid gland is a deficiency in one or more of certain essential nutrients, including the following:

- Iodine: An essential element for the formation of thyroid hormones.

- L-Tyrosine: An amino acid that is also an essential element the thyroid requires in order to produce hormones.

- Zinc

- Selenium

- Vitamin A

- Iron

With the exception of Iodine, it's probably best to get these nutrients from foods that contain them, though I do recommend fulvic minerals as a trace mineral supplement. Iodine supplements are a good idea but proceed with caution. You do not want to get too much iodine.

Hormone replacement (HRT):

Thyroid hormone replacement does not fix the problem, it does not assist the thyroid to start functioning normally, it only provides the hormones (usually only one of the hormones) that the thyroid no longer produces enough of. If you go that route, keep in mind there are physicians who believe there are better options than levothyroxine (synthetic T4). There are bioidentical thyroid hormone products that not only contain the hormones in their natural form but also contain T3, another essential thyroid hormone.

Thyroid Testing

It is a common practice in the medical community to do blood tests for one or two hormones and based on the result, prescribe levothyroxine (Synthroid), which is a synthetic copy of one of the hormones normally produced by the thyroid. In most cases, the patient will be taking levothyroxine for the rest of their life.

Many doctors test only TSH (thyroid stimulating hormone), when checking for thyroid dysfunction. TSH is not a thyroid hormone, but it is an important indicator of thyroid function. The problem is that many physicians consider TSH* to be the ultimate thyroid test and therefore use it as a stand-alone test or, in some cases, combine it with T4. However, in order to make a true, in-depth thyroid assessment a number of other tests are needed. If you really want to know what's going on with your thyroid, you may want to find a physician who will perform an array of tests, including the following:

- TSH

- T4

- T3

- Free T3

- Reverse T3

- TPO and TG (these will test for autoimmune diseases like Hashimoto's and Grave's disease.)

- Ferritin (needed to convert thyroid hormones.)

There are other tests that your doctor may wish to perform in order to have a better idea of not only what your thyroid is up to but what is going on with other endocrine glands (such as the adrenals). These glands can affect the thyroid and interact with it in what is known as the dance of the hormones.

Hashimoto's disease (AKA Hashimoto's thyroiditis):

Hashimoto's is an autoimmune disease and should be treated as such. I will write another article on autoimmune disease, but for the present, if you have Hashimoto's thyroiditis, I suggest you read my article on LDN (Low Dose Naltrexone)

There are many naturopathic physicians and functional medicine doctors who deal competently in the realm of testing for and treating thyroid issues. And there is a growing number of medical physicians who are breaking free from the archaic method of simply testing TSH and prescribing Levothyroxine. It may require a bit of searching, but you should be able to find someone.

Dr. Curtis

* Physicians and scientists cannot even agree on what is the normal range for TSH.

Chapter Eight

Much-Ignored Tragedy of Candidiasis

There is a tragedy occurring every minute of every day in our society. It causes untold deaths and enormous suffering, and it never makes the news. Few people know about it, and even fewer health professionals treat it or even attempt to do so, and those few are, for the most part, frustrated in their attempts. Some victims of this plague, mostly women, are aware they have it and try, on their own, to deal with it, but generally fail.

The villain in this scenario goes by more than one name: yeast, fungus, thrush, Candida. It is the fungal infection, Candida Albicans. And it is far more prevalent than most people, or even health professionals realize—and far more dangerous.

Candida Albicans is often the unrecognized culprit in any number of diseases.

I will name just a few: Fibromyalgia, chronic fatigue syndrome, cancer, autoimmune disease, type 2 diabetes, and many others. It is the recognized culprit in yeast infections and thrush, but it resists almost all attempts to eradicate it through conventional methods.

Carrying around trillions of microscopic fungal organisms in one's body isn't the real cause of the diseases that result from candida; it's the toxins these organisms produce. A tiny fungal cell has a very short lifespan. During that lifespan, it produces exotoxins, and when it dies, its cell wall ruptures and releases endotoxins. These toxins cause a wide array of diseases in the body.

People who suffer from candida overgrowth are walking poison factories.

This is one of the reasons why detoxification is so crucial in such cases. It is also the reason why any treatment that kills candida causes a die-off reaction called the Herxheimer reaction. Symptoms of Herxheimer can be any or all of the following: Flu-like symptoms, headache, fever, skin irritation, nausea, lethargy, joint and muscle pain, sore throat, fatigue, irritability, abdominal symptoms i.e. cramps and diarrhea, and others.

Candida die-off is not fun, but later in this article, I will tell you how to minimize it.

I will also discuss effective ways to deal with candida, but first, let's discuss causes.

Causes of Candidiasis

We all have some candida organisms in our bodies, but under normal circumstances, they are too few to do us harm. But, when overgrowth occurs, the problems begin. About 80 percent of our immune system resides in the intestinal tract. This is called the intestinal biome, and it consists of large numbers of different strains of beneficial bacteria. Among the many functions of these 'friendly' organisms is that of keeping pathogenic organisms like candida from becoming too numerous. Anything that kills off significant amounts of these beneficial bacteria creates a condition called dysbiosis and clears the way for candida (and others) to begin multiplying and taking over, creating their biofilms and releasing large amounts of toxins.

There are other areas in the body where beneficial bacteria also reside, like the vagina and the mouth, and just as the intestinal biome is crucial to intestinal health and our general health, the vaginal and oral biomes are crucial to the health of their respective areas. Research has shown that the health of the vaginal biome affects the health of the entire pelvic area, and the health of the oral biome can affect the health of the entire body. More than 700 species of bacteria have been identified as living in the mouth, most of them beneficial. And according to research published in the publication Microbiome on Nov. 30, 2023, there are 28 main species and 135 subspecies of bacteria common to the vagina.

The more we learn about the bacteria that live within us and, indeed, are part of us, the more we realize how essential they are to health and longevity. We need to take care of them so they can take care of us.

Some common causes of destruction of the intestinal biome are:

- Some medications, such as antibiotics, corticosteroids, birth control pills, and others. (remember many commercial dairy, fish, and meat products contain antibiotics that were administered to the animal, bird, or fish during its life).

- Chlorinated water

- Junk foods with all their chemicals and lack of nutrients

- Failure to eat the proper foods that nourish and replenish the beneficial bacteria.

- Alcohol

- Tobacco

- Pesticides and chemicals in foods

- Artificial sweeteners (maybe)

- Stress

- Poor sleep habits

- Not enough exercise

In other words; the modern diet and lifestyle. All the things that cause so many diseases that are so prevalent in our modern world.

A few of the diseases that have been associated with destruction of the intestinal microbiota are:

- Colitis

- Irritable bowel disease

- Other gastrointestinal inflammatory diseases

- Autoimmune diseases

- Intestinal hyperpermeability (leaky gut) (which can cause a host of diseases). It is this leaky gut condition that allows candida spores to pass through the protective mucus membrane into the bloodstream and colonize other parts of the body.

- SIBO (small intestine bacterial overgrowth)

- Gynecological disorders (the gut biome has a great impact on the vaginal biome)

- Systemic candidiasis

- Hormonal issues (the gut biome is considered to be a full-fledged endocrine organ)

- Metabolic conditions (like diabetes)

- Respiratory diseases

- Neurological conditions

- Neurological conditions

- Cardiovascular conditions

- Much More

A recent article in the scientific journal Frontiers in Cellular and Infection Microbiology states the following: Recent studies suggest a potential connection between certain gut bacteria and female reproductive tract disorders, such as bacterial vaginosis (BV), cervical and endometrial cancer, polycystic ovary syndrome (PCOS), postmenopausal syndrome, endometriosis, endometritis, and uterine fibroids (UFs)

In other words, the health (or disease) of the gut microbiome affects every part of the body.

If you want to live a long and healthy life, take care of your gut!

The Oral Biome

There has been a great deal of research in recent years, showing us how important it is to maintain a healthy oral microbiome. There are even oral probiotic products available online and in health food stores.

Common causes of destruction of the oral biome (the beneficial bacteria in the mouth) include:

- Antibiotics

- Mouthwashes

- Most toothpastes (there are safe, natural toothpastes available)

- Fluoride

- Chlorine

- Antibiotics and some other medications

- Alcohol

- Tobacco

- And most of the things that also kill the beneficial bacteria in the intestines.

- A few of the diseases that may result from the destruction of the beneficial bacteria in the mouth are:

- Diseases of the oral cavity

- Cardiovascular disease

- Endocarditis (infection of the inner part of the heart)

- Pneumonia

- Complications of pregnancy and birth

- Many more

- The vaginal biome

- Common causes of destruction of the vaginal biome are:

- Some medications, like antibiotics and corticosteroids

- Douching

- Nylon underwear

- Tight pants, such as yoga pants

- Some soaps, like anti-bacterial soaps and heavily perfumed soaps

- Smoking

- Some IUDs

- Some sexual practices

- Bad nutritional habits

- A few of the problems that may result from the destruction of the beneficial, protective bacteria of the vagina are:

- Yeast infection (vaginal candidiasis)

- Bacterial vaginosis (BV)

- Any number of gynecological conditions

Keep in mind that if you have vaginal dysbiosis/candidiasis, it's almost certain you have intestinal dysbiosis/candidiasis and probably systemic candidiasis. Therefore, treatment should not be simply targeted at the vaginal issue.

Uterine Biome

Yes, recent research has shown that though it has long been believed that the uterus is a sterile organ, there are microorganisms in there. Furthermore, in some women, the uterine microbiota is different from the vaginal microbiota. Viruses, bacteria, and at least one type of yeast have been found to be normal, non-pathogenic components of the uterine biome in both pregnant and non-pregnant women. It is now believed that alterations in the composition of the uterine biome can affect fertility.

Hormonal changes can have an effect on the uterine biome.

There is no aspect of our health that is not affected, negatively or positively, by the microorganisms that are so much a part of us that they can be considered another organ. We are a collection of different types of cells; skin, bone, muscle, nerve, mucosal, etc.—and microorganisms. Collectively, many liver cells comprise a complete liver. Collectively, many cells of different types comprise all the organs and parts of the body. Collectively, the living microorganisms comprise another organ that is our biome, a living, functioning, and essential part of us. And, if we look at all the physiologic functions that depend on our biome and are affected by it, it may be safe to say that it is the most important organ we possess. And when that organ is weakened or compromised in any way, the result is disease or even death.

Enter Candida Albicans, a destructive fungus.

Systemic candidiasis is extremely common in Western society, but rarely diagnosed. Many people have it without being aware they do. When candidiasis causes disease, in most cases the disease (or its symptoms) is treated, but nothing is done for the candidiasis, which is at the root of the problem.

It would be nice if a simple antifungal medication could eradicate candida from the body. But, while there are prescription medications that have some limited effectiveness, a simple antifungal, whether it is a prescription medication or a natural substance, only addresses one aspect of a multifaceted problem and is destined to fail.

Natural remedies for candida abound, and most of them, like the medical antifungals, have some effect, but in the end, the fungus always seems to triumph. The main reason for this is that candida forms defensive biofilms that protect it from the immune system and antifungals, be they medical or natural.

What is the solution?

Let's divide this answer into two parts: The solution for avoiding candida and the solution for fixing the problem of candida overgrowth.

It needs to be understood that there are always some candida organisms in the body, but a normal biome and a well-functioning immune system keep them in check. When something causes large-scale destruction to our beneficial, protective bacteria, the candida is allowed to grow and spread out of control. These beneficial bacteria constitute at least 80 percent of the internal army that protects us from attack from without and from within

Antibiotics are a huge part of the problem.

It's true antibiotics can and often do, save lives, but it's the opinion of many researchers that they are very much overused. Increasing numbers of medical providers are trying to be more conservative in prescribing antibiotics, but the problem is not a simple one to fix. This is an area in which natural medicine excels.

Most of the things that are destructive to the protective bacteria that comprise our biome; things like junk food, alcohol, tobacco, chlorine, and many others, can be avoided, and the individual will benefit in many ways if they are.

How to fix your candidiasis.

There are as many approaches to this problem as there are opinions. And for every opinion, there are a hundred natural candida cleanses, candida clears, candida fighters, killers, and what-have-yous sold in health food stores and online. Obviously, I haven't seen them all in action, but the ones I've seen haven't impressed me.

Most of them have some good ingredients, but they are inadequate. They don't address all the many complex aspects of dysbiosis and candidiasis.

I don't claim to have all the answers, I don't believe anyone does, nor could anyone possibly scrutinize all the mountains of scientific literature on this subject, but, if you suffer from this problem, I am confident I can give you some information that will help.

Candidiasis is fixable, but it requires a multipronged approach.

The dysbiosis has to be addressed, the biofilms have to be eliminated, the candida organisms have to be killed, and successive generations of fungi hatched from the eggs left by the previous generation also have to be killed off, each generation becoming less numerous than the last; the body has to be cleansed, the intestinal hyperpermeability has to be corrected, and the immune system has to be strengthened. Additionally, the individual has to change the habits that have allowed the problem to grow and continue.

See what I meant when I said it is a complex solution?

How to minimize die-off (Herxheimer) reaction.

Before you begin a candida program, be prepared for the inevitable die-off reaction. It usually lasts from 3 days to a week, and can be minimized by the following:

- Drink a lot of purified water

- Coconut charcoal: 1 or 2 capsules 3 times daily. This will adsorb many of the impurities in the intestinal tract that are created by the die-off of the candida and keep them from entering the blood.

- Enzymes: My preferred product for this purpose is Flavenzyme from vitacost.com. Dosage: 7 tablets first thing in the morning on an empty stomach with 16 oz of purified water. Don't eat anything for 1½ to 2 hours, but continue drinking water every ½ hour until you eat. Do the same in the afternoon or evening if you can arrange to have an empty stomach. Taken this way, the enzymes will be very beneficial in cleansing the blood and minimizing the Herxheimer reaction. The enzymes will also play a crucial role in breaking down the biofilms that protect the candida organisms.

Killing Candida

To eradicate candida, you must destroy its strongholds. Its biofilms.

The following is a list of natural substances that have been shown in scientific studies to eliminate biofilms and/or kill candida albicans. (Please understand that everyone has different needs, so the dosages in the lists below are guidelines only). I have divided the list into two categories: the substances that break down biofilms and also kill candida organisms, and those that kill candida but do not affect the biofilms.

Natural antifungals shown scientifically to also eradicate biofilms:

- **Enzymes. My preferred product for this purpose is, again, Flavenzyme from vitacost.com. (mentioned above) Dosage: 7 tablets first thing in the morning on an empty stomach, with 16 oz of purified water. Don't eat anything for 1½ to 2 hours, but continue drinking water every ½ hour until you eat. Do the same in the afternoon or evening if you can arrange to have an empty stomach.

- **Xylitol A natural, healthy sugar. (and, yes, diabetics can take it.)

- Eucalyptus oil ½ ml to 2 ml daily.

- *NAC (N acetyl Cysteine) 200 to 600 mg 3 times daily.

- Colloidal silver: I prefer ionic silver (ACS 200 from Results RNA)

- **Coconut oil (virgin, organic) 1 tablespoonful 3 times daily.

- **Citrus Pectin 10-20 grams daily

- *Berberine 500 mg 2 or 3 times daily.

- EGCG. Start with 200 mg 2 times daily, build up over 1 month to 400 mg 2 times daily.

- *Oregano oil (Wld, Mediterranean) 1 drop in water 3 times daily. Build up to 2 drops 3 times daily.

- *Piperine 5 mg 3 times daily.

- *Undecylenic acid 250 mg 3 times daily.

- Grapefruit seed extract 10-12 drops in water 2 or 3 times daily.

- Natural antifungals that kill candida but may not break down biofilms:

- *Food-grade diatomaceous earth 1 tsp one time daily, build up over 10 days to 1 tsp 2 times daily in water. Do not inhale. Must be food grade!

- *Olive leaf extract 500 mg 2 times daily

- **Prebiotics

- **Probiotics

- **Fermented foods (essential)

I would not recommend trying to take everything on the above lists at once.

I have placed a star next to the ones I have chosen as the primary ones. They are all excellent, but the non-starred ones are optional. You may even want to alternate, taking the single-starred ones one week and the non-starred ones the next. The ones with 2 stars should be taken regardless of what else is taken.

Butyrate

Nothing is more important than butyrate, for gut health and the health of the beneficial bacteria in the gut. In a normal gut or a diseased gut, butyrate is essential. It is also essential in dealing with candidiasis and with the leaky gut issue that is commonly associated with it. Below is a list of butyrate-producing foods. The term butyrate-producing foods means they are foods that feed the bacteria in the gut that produce butyrate.

- Honey (MUST BE raw, organic, unprocessed).

- Sweet potato

- Zucchini

- Cruciferous vegetables

- Purple kale.

- Purple cabbage.

- Eggplant.

- Radish.

- Green banana (organic) (must be VERY GREEN), or you can buy green banana powder as a supplement.

The Diet

An important aspect of killing candida involves starving the fungal organisms.

For in-depth nutritional recommendations, I recommend the website   Their candida diet is healthy, and it will keep the candida from having any food source. They even have an e-book with candida-friendly recipes.

Good luck, friends, and be patient. It takes months.

Chapter Nine

Leaky Gut - You May Have It - Here's How to Fix It If You Do

It was sometime in the 1970s when I first read the statement attributed to Hippocrates, "All disease begins in the gut." I didn't believe it. I couldn't understand how that could be the case. Now, after nearly 50 years of health research and clinical work, I recognize that, with a few exceptions, that statement is one of the most powerful statements: one of the most significant truths in the realm of human health.

If you want to live a long and healthy life, you must own that concept. You must not only believe it, but you must also understand WHY it is true. If you do not if you are scratching your head at this moment, trying to grasp this thing, don't feel bad. You are not alone. I will do my best in this article to give you a solid understanding of this crucial truth.

Where to begin?

I could begin with a discussion of the importance of nutrition in our health. In fact, nutrition is undoubtedly the most important subject regarding human health (and the most neglected in our society).

Or I could begin by discussing what is quite possibly our most important organ, the intestinal biome, which is, ironically, our most neglected organ. In fact, most people, including health professionals, don't even view it as an organ.

I could also approach the subject by discussing the importance of the function and health of the intestinal mucosal barrier (AKA intestinal barrier AKA mucosal barrier) in human health and longevity and how disease (or health) begins there.

But let's begin--appropriately–at birth. A child, we'll call her Jane, is in the womb. Her gastrointestinal tract is sterile. She has no biome. In other words, there are no microorganisms in her entire G.I. tract. As she passes through the birth canal to begin her mortal sojourn, microorganisms that are present in her mother's vagina enter Jane's mouth. And her microbiome is initialized.

What is leaky gut syndrome?

The intestinal lining (called the mucosa) is lined with a protective layer of specialized cells that are linked together by proteins called tight junction proteins. These tight junctions control what passes from the intestines into the blood. Their job is to ensure that toxins, pathogenic bacteria, and other things that do not belong in our blood do not pass through. But they do allow essential substances like nutrients to pass unopposed. This is called selective permeability.

When these tight junctions are compromised, the intestinal mucosa becomes too permeable (intestinal hyperpermeability or leaky gut) and serious health problems are unavoidable. The harmful proteins, toxins, antigens, and pathogenic organisms that then cross over into the bloodstream are at the root of many diseases that we know of and undoubtedly many that have not yet been conclusively proven to result from leaky gut.

The following is a partial list of conditions that have been attributed to leaky gut syndrome.

- Bowel diseases (IBS, Crohn's, ulcerative colitis, etc.)

- Arthritis

- Autoimmune diseases (M.S, lupus, Hashimoto's, rheumatoid arthritis, many more)

- Chronic and acute inflammatory conditions (too numerous to list)

- Obesity and other metabolic diseases (like type 2 diabetes, fatty liver, and more)

- Fibromyalgia

- Weakened immune system (this can result in a host of health problems)

- Chronic fatigue syndrome

- Asthma

- Some neurological disorders (like Parkinson's)

- Colorectal cancer

- Esophageal cancer

- Probably other cancers as well

- Blood disorders

- Hormonal issues

- Acne and other skin conditions

- Thyroid disorders

- Celiac disease

- Gluten intolerance

- Diarrhea

- Nutritional deficiencies (due to malabsorption)

- Many types of infectious conditions

- Allergies (seasonal and food-related)

- Much more

So, it appears old Hippocrates was right. If you look at the list above it would seem that just about any disease can (and probably does) originate in the gut, either directly or indirectly.

Leaky gut/intestinal hyperpermeability is a controversial subject in the medical community. Some doctors don't believe in it, others see it as a gray area, and still others say they believe in intestinal hyperpermeability, but not in leaky gut, (as though they were two different things). Meanwhile, they continue treating the symptoms of the diseases related to leaky gut, with drugs that, in some cases, are the very ones that caused the problem (or contributed to it) to begin with.

To my knowledge, there is no effective medical treatment for this problem. The methods that truly work are all natural. And, as always in the natural realm of healing, the first starting point is to discontinue doing/consuming the things that caused the problem to begin with, or that interfere with correcting it. So let's talk about those.

Causes of leaky gut syndrome

Dysbiosis. It is my opinion that dysbiosis is the number one factor in leaky gut syndrome. This occurs when the intestinal biome is damaged (as with antibiotic use). The normal biome consists of many different strains of beneficial microorganisms. It is a living community of living organisms, each of which contributes different things to the community and the normal functioning of the body and the brain.

Below is a list of some of the things that can cause dysbiosis. Many of the things on the list can damage the intestinal mucosa in other ways, in addition to causing dysbiosis.

Some common causes of destruction of the intestinal biome are:

Some medications, such as antibiotics, corticosteroids, birth control pills, and others. (remember, many commercial dairy, fish, and meat products contain antibiotics that were administered to the animal, bird, or fish during its life. (Another reason to eat organic)

- Chlorinated water

- Junk foods with all their chemicals and lack of nutrients

- Failure to eat the proper foods that nourish and replenish the beneficial bacteria

- Alcohol

- Tobacco

- Pesticides and chemicals in foods

- Artificial sweeteners (maybe)

- Stress

- Candida Albicans (See my article on Candidiasis)

- Poor sleep habits

- Insufficient exercise

- Chronic constipation

- In other words; the modern diet and lifestyle. Many of the things that cause so many diseases that are so prevalent in our modern world.

A few of the diseases that have been associated with dysbiosis (damaged intestinal microbiota) are:

- Colitis

- Irritable bowel disease

- Other gastrointestinal inflammatory diseases

- Autoimmune diseases

- Intestinal hyperpermeability (leaky gut)

- SIBO (small intestine bacterial overgrowth)

- Gynecological disorders (the gut biome has a great impact on the vaginal biome)

- Systemic candidiasis

- Hormonal issues (the gut biome is considered to be a full-fledged endocrine organ)

- Metabolic conditions (like diabetes)

- Respiratory diseases

- Neurological conditions

- Neurological conditions

- Cardiovascular conditions

- Much More

A recent article in the scientific journal, Frontiers in Cellular and Infection Microbiology states the following: Recent studies suggest a potential connection between certain gut bacteria and female reproductive tract disorders, such as bacterial vaginosis (BV), cervical and endometrial cancer, polycystic ovary syndrome (PCOS), post-menopausal syndrome, endometriosis, endometritis, and uterine fibroids (UFs)

In other words, the health (or disease) of the gut microbiome affects every part of the body.

So, what can be done about leaky gut syndrome?

Avoid the following things:

Healing the gut requires a multifaceted approach, the obvious first step of which is to avoid the things that caused the problem to begin with. See the partial list of those things, below.

- Sugar (including high fructose corn syrup and agave)

- Pasteurized dairy products. (butter is healthy. Avoid butter substitutes)

- Gluten

- Chlorinated water.

- Seed oils (vegetable oils)

- Junk foods with all their chemicals and lack of nutrients

- Low fiber diet

- Failure to eat the proper foods that nourish and replenish the beneficial bacteria.

- Alcohol

- Tobacco

- Pesticides and chemicals in foods

- Artificial sweeteners (maybe)

- Harmful beverages like soda, energy drinks, sports drinks, and others. These harm health in numerous ways.

Certain medications cause dysbiosis by killing the microbiota

Antibiotics, for example, don't know when to stop killing. They kill the good bacteria along with the bad. However, If you are taking a prescribed medication, consult a qualified healthcare professional before stopping. Don't try to do it alone.

Re-establish the intestinal biome

Once the individual has eliminated the causative factors, they need to begin re-establishing the intestinal biome. Below are some recommendations for accomplishing that.

Butyrate

Nothing is more important than butyrate for gut health and the health of the beneficial bacteria in the gut. In a normal gut or a diseased gut, butyrate is essential. It is also essential in dealing with leaky gut syndrome. Below is a list of butyrate-producing foods. The term butyrate-producing foods means they are foods that feed the bacteria in the gut that produce butyrate.

- Vegetable fiber - Eat lots of fresh, raw organic vegetables.

- Honey (MUST BE raw, organic, unprocessed).

- Sweet potato

- Zucchini

- Cruciferous vegetables

- Purple kale.

- Purple cabbage.

- Eggplant.

- Radish.

- Green banana (organic) (must be VERY GREEN), or you can buy green banana powder as a supplement.

- Probiotics, prebiotics, and fermented foods. These are essential for replenishing the intestinal biome. Many people think they can simply eat some yogurt, and it will do the job.

It won't.

Kill candida

If there is a problem with candidiasis, the candida needs to be gotten under control. This is not easily done, mostly due to the biofilms the candida organism constructs to protect itself. For information on candidiasis and how to eliminate it and its biofilms, see my article on that subject.

Avoid constipation!

Constipation is much more than just a minor annoyance; it is potentially very harmful to the health and very damaging to the colon and the intestinal microbiota.

Detoxify and heal the colon

A few of the things that can help with colon detox and regeneration are:

- Drinking a lot of purified water.

- Drinking 2 large glasses of warm, purified water first thing in the morning on an empty stomach. Then, if possible don't eat anything for ½ hour or more. This is a powerful healing remedy for the colon, the rest of the G.I. tract, the liver, and the kidneys. The water should be warmed on the stove, not in a microwave. Do not drink tap water.

- Coconut charcoal - 1 or 2 capsules 3 times daily. This will adsorb many of the impuriaies in the intestinal tract, and keep them from entering the blood.

- Psyllium fiber - (Pronounced silly um) 2 to 4 tablespoons in a glass of water at bedtime.

- Juicing - fresh, raw, organic vegetables (not fruit)

- Fermented foods - This is crucial!

- L-Glutamine - This is an amino acid that is very beneficial to the colon. 5,000 - 10,000 mg daily is a common dosage.

- Aloe vera

- Slippery elm

- Coconut oil

- Butyrate - I mention butyrate again because it is so important. Remember, the key is not to eat butyrate-containing foods but to eat foods that feed the bacteria in the gut that produce butyrate. A list of those is provided above.

- Herbs

- There are a number of herbs that are beneficial in colon cleansing. Below is a partial list.

- Aloe vera

- Ginger

- Turmeric (use fresh turmeric root, or make sure your product is lead-free

- Dandelion root

- Licorice root

- Fennel

- Mint

- Lemongrass

I truly believe Hippocrates was right. And, if we don't take care of our gut health, we will leave ourselves at risk for almost any disease. The more we learn about the gut and its relation to general health, the more we recognize the need to care for it. And the more we learn about the bacteria that live within us and, indeed, are part of us, the more we realize how essential they are to health and longevity. We need to take care of them so they can take care of us.

Chapter Ten

Science-Based Natural Medicine for a Healthy Heart

N othing makes a person happier than having a happy heart."

Roy T. Bennet

Two huge issues that all humans face are:

1. Our lives depend on our hearts. If the heart stops, we stop. End of story.

2. The modern diet and lifestyle are heart killers.

We are having an obesity epidemic. We are having a cancer epidemic. We are having a diabetes epidemic. We are having a heart disease epidemic.

And they all have the same causes: The modern diet and lifestyle.

I won't belabor that issue too much in this article, because I have written about it in numerous other articles. Suffice it to say that a diet laden with sugar, seed oils, addictive chemicals like caffeine, monosodium glutamate, chemical sweeteners, genetically modified foods, pesticides, processed junk foods, and very few micronutrients is at the root of it all. (I should mention, as well, that people who smoke, drink, vape, and do drugs are at much higher risk of heart disease than those who take care of their hearts).

But, enough about that. In this article, I will discuss science-based, natural ways to keep a healthy heart healthy as well as things that are used to restore an ailing heart to normal function.

"Ah, Nothing is too late, till the tired heart shall cease to palpitate."

Henry Wadsworth Longfellow

Healing the heart is an area in which natural medicine excels.

Nature has provided us with numerous heart healers. So many, in fact, that the challenge often is choosing from all the good options.

There are, however, certain natural medicines that, in my opinion, are a good idea in almost every case. These are:

- Cayenne (AKA capsicum)

- Hawthorn berry

- Magnesium Taurate

- Taurine (an amino acid)

- Omega 3 fatty acids

- D-Ribose

- CoQ10

- Garlic

- Vitamin K2 (AKA K2,7 or menaquinone)

- Water - Drinking plenty of pure water is very important for heart health.

Important!

There is an issue that is often encountered by patients who are attempting to heal their hearts using natural medicines. Many times, these individuals have been under medical care and are taking blood thinning medications. In these cases, some of the most effective natural medicines are contraindicated, as they may also have a blood-thinning effect. If you are taking blood thinners, you should consult a qualified healthcare professional before taking any natural medicine that may create a negative interaction.

When blood viscosity is in an abnormal state, events such as abnormal clot formation, strokes, and other hazards related to blood abnormalities can occur. Fortunately, there are natural ways to normalize blood viscosity. (I don't care for the term 'blood thinner' in reference to these natural healing agents because they do not artificially thin the blood. Blood thinning medications create an unnatural and potentially dangerous situation in which the normal blood clotting mechanism is compromised, whereas the natural substances have the effect of, as mentioned above, normalizing the blood in terms of viscosity, clotting ability, and other factors. Normal blood does not behave in an abnormal way).

The importance of normal blood viscosity cannot be overstated. Much depends on it, including the health and longevity of the heart. Perhaps the most common cause of hyper viscosity of the blood is simply not drinking enough water. Notice I didn't use the word 'fluid'. I said water. The human body is designed to drink water—a lot of it. Some beverages dehydrate, as opposed to hydrating.

Below is a list of natural substances that have been shown to possess the property of normalizing blood viscosity.

- Vitamin E

- Turmeric (make sure it is lead-free)

- Cayenne (Capsicum)

- Ginger root

- Garlic

- Ginkgo biloba

- Omega 3 fatty acids

- Water - I mention it again because it is so important.

Take a moment to thank your heart. Think about what it has to do. It is a hollow muscle that has to alternately contract and relax unceasingly 24 hours a day, 365 days a year for your entire life—without stopping!

E.B. White said, "I am reminded of the advice of my neighbor. Never worry about your heart till it stops beating."

Bad advice. We should think of our heart health every day, with everything we put into our body, every time we exercise or don't exercise when we should. Every time we are tempted to do something we know to be harmful to the heart, we should think of that organ, what it does, and where we would be if it stopped doing it.

Chapter Eleven

Polycystic Ovary Syndrome (PCOS)

One of the areas in which scientific, natural medicine excels is in dealing with Polycystic ovary syndrome (often called polycystic ovarian syndrome), or PCOS.

I need to begin this article with a brief discussion of philosophy—more precisely, conventional medical philosophy versus natural medicine philosophy.

What I'm about to say is in no way intended to be a criticism of anyone or any profession. I will merely state certain obvious facts:

Medical professionals often label diseases as being "incurable" or having "no known cure" simply because they have no cure for them.

Medical professionals often make statements like "the cause is unknown", simply because they do not know the cause.

In these statements, the fact that there are proven, scientific natural treatments, methods, and knowledge is completely disregarded. As though they simply did not exist.

I would prefer they would say something like the following: "We, those of us who practice and study allopathic (conventional) medicine, do not have a cure, or we do not know the cause of your disorder, but there are other methods, other healthcare professions, other realms of knowledge.

But they almost never do.

My reason for writing the above is that in conventional medicine, the cause of PCOS is considered to be unknown, and there is considered to be no cure.

I disagree.

I am not criticizing; I am simply offering an alternative approach to a very serious problem, and I will repeat the statement with which I began this article:

One of the areas in which scientific, natural medicine excels is in dealing with Polycystic ovary syndrome (often called polycystic ovarian syndrome), or PCOS.

Having said that, let's get down to business.

How do you know if you have PCOS? It's usually quite easy to spot because there are numerous external signs of the condition (aside from the ovarian cysts for which the condition is named). Below is a list of signs to check for:

- Abnormal menstrual periods: Irregular periods, heavy bleeding, missed periods.

- Infertility: It is claimed that PCOS is the most common cause of female infertility.

- Obesity: Not all women with PCOS will have a weight problem, but many do.

- Acne: Especially on the face, chest, and back.

- Abnormal hair growth: (hirsutism) This can be on the face, arms, chest, or abdomen. This results from increased levels of male hormones called androgens.

- Ovarian cysts or enlarged ovaries.

- Thinning hair: Balding, or hair loss in patches.

- Areas of darker skin: (acanthosis nigricans) Commonly in the armpits, groin area, under the breasts, and the folds of the neck.

- Skin tags: Small flaps of skin, sometimes found all over the body, most commonly on the neck and in the armpits.

Keep in mind, however, that it is possible to have PCOS without having any observable outward symptoms.

There is a strong correlation between insulin resistance and PCOS. And, of course, insulin resistance can result in type ll diabetes and metabolic syndrome, which includes heart disease, stroke, and a few other very undesirable and very serious health conditions.

It has been considered for years that PCOS is a risk factor for developing type 2 diabetes; however, it makes sense that it is the insulin resistance that causes the PCOS (see my article on insulin resistance).

Having mentioned insulin, we have entered the realm of hormones. I have written articles about leptin (a hormone) resistance, insulin (another hormone) resistance, and the human biome, which is now considered by many researchers to be, among many other things, another organ—specifically, an endocrine (hormonal) organ (see my article on leaky gut).

They all work together. And when one is affected., they all are affected. When one of them becomes dysfunctional, there is a domino effect that causes a cascade of symptoms resulting in things like—well PCOS, among others.

True healing is only done by the body. No person heals another person. And, true healing involves treating the body, not the disease, and certainly not the symptoms of the disease. It is essential to understand these things if we are to assist the body in correcting malfunctions.

In order to assist the body in healing itself of diseases like the ones listed above, the nutritional causes of those issues must be addressed.

So, by way of preventing degenerative diseases, including insulin resistance, you may want to consider the following:

Things to avoid

- Avoid all beverages except the healthy ones: herbal teas (no caffeine, please), fresh juice from raw, organic vegetables (not fruit. Eating fruit is great, drinking them is not), and water; the one beverage our bodies were designed to drink.

- Avoid sugar or cut down to occasional, small amounts. It is my belief that insulin resistance is primarily a nutritional disease and that the two primary nutritional factors are seed oils (vegetable oils) and sugar (including high fructose corn syrup and agave). You can substitute with organic, raw, unprocessed honey, monk fruit (without erythritol), or stevia (pure, nothing else added) in limited amounts. (again, fruits are healthy, drinking fruit juices is not).

- Avoid chemical (artificial) sweeteners. There are a number of studies linking artificial sweeteners to insulin resistance.

- Avoid vegetable (seed) oils (canola oil, soy oil, corn oil, sunflower oil, safflower oil, cottonseed oil, rice bran oil, grape-

seed oil), and replace them with coconut oil, avocado oil, *
olive oil, * beef tallow, butter, ghee. You will also have a much
easier time losing weight if you replace the vegetable oils with
the recommendable oils.

- Avoid monosodium glutamate (MSG) (see my article on this
subject)

- Do I need to tell you that you need to avoid alcohol, tobacco,
and illicit drugs? I didn't think so.

The Lists

You will not be able to take all the things on the following lists, nor
should you try. Each individual has different needs, and I have no way
of knowing what yours are.

Some people (generally those with a weight problem) will need
to deal with leptin resistance, first. Then they may find that other
problems, such as insulin resistance, will have been resolved. Others
will need to address the insulin resistance, followed by the PCOS.
Some people will need to address their leaky gut to begin with, and
others will find that they may attack the PCOS directly.

I have posted articles on this newsletter platform dealing in depth
with the above-mentioned subjects. If you wish to take charge of your
health, you can read those articles and tailor the information in them
to your individual needs.

It may seem a bit overwhelming, but I believe you will find that
as you begin to create your individualized program, things will just
seem to fall into place. It's not as hard as it may seem. This newsletter
with its many articles and features has been meticulously designed to
assist people like you, beginner or expert, or anywhere in between in
acquiring the information and skills needed for a long and healthy life.

The following is a list of things that have been shown scientifically to benefit individuals with PCOS, along with dosages that have been used:

- Inositol (Myo and D-Chiro in a 40-1 ratio): 2,000 to 4,000 mg daily

- Tribulus Terrestris: 750 to 1200 mg daily

- Ceylon cinnamon: 500 to 3,000 mg daily

- Licorice Root: Depends on the product. Follow label instructions.

- Silymarin: 200 to 400 mg daily

- Fenugreek: 1,000 to 5,000 mg daily

- Peony: Follow label instructions

- Black Cohosh: Depends on the product. Follow label instructions

- St. John's wort: 300 mg daily

- If you have a weight problem, you may want to read my article on weight control, in which I discuss leptin resistance, among many other things.

Leptin Resistance

Leptin resistance can cause numerous health problems, including obesity and insulin resistance (which can cause PCOS and obesity).

The following is a list of things that have been shown scientifically to reduce leptin resistance, along with dosages that have been used:

- Fulvic acid. No dosage has been established

- Colostrum. Follow product recommendations

- Alpha lipoic acid. 600 to 1800 mg daily

- Berberine. 500 mg 2 or 3 times daily

- GAG (glycosaminoglycans). Follow label recommendations

- Zinc. 25 mg daily

- Soluble fiber (like Psyllium)

- Fish oil. 3,000 to 9,000 mg daily

- Get plenty of sleep. Very important!

Insulin Resistance

The following is a list of some of the things that have been shown scientifically to reduce insulin resistance along with dosages that have been used:

- Magnesium Glycinate. At least 420 mg daily

- Fulvic acid. No dosage has been established.

- Glycine. An amino acid. 4,000 mg daily to 8,000 mg daily, with food

- N-acetylcysteine (NAC). Also an amino acid. 400 mg to 1,000 mg daily, with food.

- Neem oil. Take as directed on the label.

- Cat's claw. 300-500 mg 3 times daily

- Quercetin. 500 to 1,000 mg daily

- Resveratrol. Around 2,000 mg daily

- Bergamot. 500 to 1,000 mg daily

- Ceylon Cinnamon. 500 mg to 3,000 mg daily

- Garlic. No dosage has been established

- Berberine. 500 mg 2 or 3 times daily

- Curcumin. 500 to 2,000 mg daily

- Vitamin D3. Be tested first to know how your levels are

- Vitamin K2,7 (AKA MK7) (AKA Menaquinone). At least 100 mcg for every 1,000 iu of D3 taken.

- Trace minerals from the sea or from the Great Salt Lake (Concentrace liquid drops). Dosage as directed.

- Juicing fresh, raw, organic vegetables (not fruit) every day.

- Lack of exercise is a big contributor to diseases like resistance to leptin and insulin.

One thing everyone agrees on is that lack of exercise contributes to insulin resistance and that obesity, especially central obesity is a huge risk marker for the condition. It is worth noting that the things that appear to be among the main causes of I.R. also cause obesity.

Intermittent fasting can help with both insulin resistance and leptin resistance.

If you have a leaky gut (intestinal hyperpermeability), you should take steps to correct that problem as well. (see my article on leaky gut)

* Not all olive oil and avocado oil products sold are pure, even if the label says extra virgin. Many companies mix their oils with harmful oils like soy and canola and do not list them on the label. For the benefit of my subscribers, on this newsletter platform, I have provided a list of some of the products that have been tested as pure.

Chapter Twelve

Healthy Liver, Healthy Life

I f I were asked to distill my approach to healing down to the two most fundamental recommendations, they would be these: Heal your liver and heal your gut.

I have written extensively about gut health (see my articles on leaky gut and candidiasis), so I will dedicate this article to that multitalented, all-important, miracle organ, the liver.

The liver is not only one of our most important organs; it is one of the most neglected. Only when blood tests show that the liver is struggling do we even take notice of the fact that we have one? Otherwise, we ignore it as it carries on its more than 500 functions (that we know of) in the body. However, some things can adversely affect the liver that does not show up on routine blood tests. In fact, there are things that can affect the liver for which we have no tests at all.

We are a society that rarely deals with causes of problems. Nor, for the most part, do we deal with prevention. We wait for a problem—in this case, a health problem—to occur and we then deal with the symptoms of the problem.

The average person takes better care of their car than their liver.

Cleansing: One Aspect of Liver Health.

Many health professionals believe the liver is perfectly able to cleanse itself and should be left alone until it begins to manifest symptoms or abnormal blood test results.

And it's true; the liver is very good at cleansing itself—under normal circumstances. But we don't live in normal circumstances. The things that assault our livers on a daily basis are, in many cases, things that through all the millennia of human existence did not even exist until recent years.

Our bodies and our livers are constantly bombarded with chemicals coming at us from all directions. They are in our water, our air, our personal products, even the clothes we wear, and the sheets, mattresses, and pillows we sleep on are full of toxic chemicals. We eat genetically modified, hybridized, denatured, synthetically enriched, microwaved garbage that doesn't even belong in the ecosystem, much less on the dinner table. Foods that have been filled with pesticides are grown in toxic soil with chemical fertilizers that create high yields and add no vitamins or minerals to the plant. And still more chemicals are added to these foods before they reach the grocery store. We eat fast foods because we are too lazy or too rushed to cook a decent meal, we eat microwaved, pre-packaged foods full of chemicals. We consume large amounts of sugar and industrial oils (seed oils), we drink water and other liquids out of plastic bottles that add even more chemicals to our bodies, or we drink tap water that is polluted with toxic chemicals, including some that we add intentionally. We have even polluted our oceans, vast as they are, so that fish that were formerly healthy to eat are now filled with poisons.

Babies are being born now with over 280 chemicals circulating in their bloodstream.

Most of us fail to eat significant quantities of natural foods that contain the substances the liver requires in order to tackle the overwhelming job of detoxification. We live in a society that attacks symptoms of disease with over the counter and prescription drugs. Our bodies are toxic waste dumps, and we wonder why we are the sickest society that has ever lived on the planet. We wonder why life expectancy is plummeting.

We wonder why degenerative diseases like cancer, type ll diabetes, heart disease, autoimmune disease, and others that were rare a hundred years ago are now merely accepted as a part of life. We wonder why obesity, with all its attendant complications, has gone from being rare 100 years ago to about 42% today (in the United States). In fact, the rate of obesity in the U.S. has tripled in the past 60 years. (keep in mind that obesity is very damaging to the liver).

Our bodies are filled with chemicals that, in most cases didn't exist a hundred years (in many cases even thirty years) ago, and then we say ridiculous things like, "The liver is perfectly capable of detoxifying itself," and we leave it to do this mountainous task with absolutely no assistance from us.

A bird preens itself every day. It requires no help in performing this routine task of personal hygiene. But imagine that same bird has been caught in an oil spill and is covered with tar from beak to feet. Nature has simply not equipped that creature to cope with such an unnatural situation.

Do you see the parallel here? Our livers need our help!

The liver is the mastermind of the body. It regulates the function of every other part of the body. It plays an essential role in the function and health of all other organs and systems. And when it is struggling, our general health can be affected. Blood tests only provide bits of information as to what is happening inside an unhealthy liver. And they don't tell us why it is happening.

Perhaps one of the reasons the liver is so ignored is because it is so amazing. Did you know that, aside from the human biome, the liver is the only organ that can fully regenerate? If two-thirds of the liver were removed, it would regrow to its original size in eight to fifteen days.

In order to gain an appreciation of the importance of the liver in human health, it is helpful to have an understanding of some of the jobs it performs. Below is a list of just a few of those over 500 functions.

Production of cholesterol: Yes, most of the cholesterol in your blood is produced by your liver. Cholesterol is essential for life and good health, and the liver makes sure we have enough for our needs—unless we interfere with that essential process.

- Immunity: The liver is an essential part of our immune system.

- Digestion: Proper liver function is essential for all aspects of digestion.

- Production and storage of glycogen: Glycogen is stored energy. The liver seems to have an almost unlimited capacity for glycogen storage.

- Production of amino acids, enzymes, urea, and albumin: These are all essential for life.

- Production of thousands of chemicals that the body requires to carry on the countless functions of life.

- Storage of micro-nutrients.

- Proper brain function.

- Hormone regulation.

- Adrenal function.

- Blood filtering and detoxification.

- Excretion of toxic substances.

The list goes on and on.

The steps that must be taken to cleanse the liver and restore it to proper function are:

1. Stop doing the things that have caused the problem! This is only common sense.

2. Cleanse the liver.

3. Repair and build the liver.

Below is a list of some of the common things that damage the liver

- Alcohol

- Tobacco

- Drugs

Illicit drugs like cocaine, heroin, methamphetamine, fentanyl, and others are very hepatotoxic (toxic to the liver). Some prescription medications can harm the liver as well. It is always a good idea to read about the side effects of your medication(s). Some medications are so dangerous to the liver that prescribers are required to conduct periodic blood tests to see how much damage has been done. One of the most popular categories of prescription medications is also one of the common causes of liver damage. These are the Statin drugs (cholesterol-lowering drugs).

An article in 2018 in Current Medical Chemistry makes the following statement: "Statins are a class of drugs whose main adverse effects are drug-induced liver injury and myopathy.

- Over-the-counter medications - Some over-the-counter medications, such as Acetaminophen (Tylenol/paracetamol), are also hepatotoxic. I will discuss this drug more in-depth later in this article.

- Sugar - By this, I mean fructose in table sugar (sucrose), high fructose corn syrup, agave, and fructose products. (fruit is fine). (See my article on sweeteners).

- Caffeine - The research on this addictive chemical is controversial. Some researchers claim it can be beneficial, while others claim it causes cancer and other diseases. Sometimes, it helps to insert common logic into the equation, so let me ask you: do you really believe that a substance as addictive as caffeine can be safe to consume day after day? Can you name a single addictive substance that is not harmful?

In a study published in 2020 by Cui WQ et al., the following introductory statement is made: "Caffeine is a purine alkaloid and is widely consumed in coffee, soda, tea, chocolate, and energy drinks. To date, a growing number of studies have indicated that caffeine is associated with many diseases, including colorectal cancer."

- Glyphosate (roundup) and other pesticides - (eat organic foods!)

- Acetaminophen/Paracetamol - I mention this drug because,

despite being an over-the-counter product, available without a prescription in any convenience store, grocery store, or gas station, it is the number one cause of liver failure in our society (surpassing even alcohol), and the top reason for which people contact the poison control center in the United States. In America, it's called Acetaminophen, in Europe, it goes by the name Paracetamol.

Many people know it as Tylenol, though it has many other trade names. Here is a list of some of them:

- Abenol

- Acephen

- APAP

- Apo-Acetaminophen

- Feverall

- Mapap

- Ofirmev

- Atasol

- Panadol

- For purposes of this article, I will refer to this drug as

Acetaminophen/Paracetamol

In addition to liver damage, Acetaminophen/paracetamol can cause kidney damage as well as some potentially fatal skin disorders. Taking it with alcohol drastically raises the risk of serious complications. Moreover, if you take just a small amount over the recommended dose of Acetaminophen/Paracetamol over a period of a few days, you put yourself at greater risk of liver damage than if you were to take one large overdose.

In a 2015 article published in the European Journal of Pain, the following statement appears, "Acetaminophen/Paracetamol is the most widely used drug in the world. At the same time, it is probably one of the most dangerous compounds in medical use..."

In an article in the Journal of Clinical and Translational Hepatology, published in June 2016, the authors make the following statement regarding the drug Acetaminophen/Paracetamol (They refer to it as APAP): "Further epidemiologic studies have demonstrated that there is a true lack of knowledge regarding the harmful potential of APAP."

Liver Cleansing

The unnatural, chemical-filled environment in which we find ourselves makes liver cleansing imperative. Fortunately, nature has provided us with many things that work very effectively for that purpose. Most of the things on the list below are also beneficial in helping the liver heal and strengthen itself, as well as maintain a healthy status.

The following is a list of some of the natural things that have been shown scientifically to cleanse (and in many cases help repair and maintain) the liver:

- Water

- Lemon juice

- Magnesium (not magnesium oxide)

- Potassium

- Alpha lipoic acid

- Choline

- N-Acetyl Cysteine (NAC)

- Zinc

- Juicing fresh, raw, organic vegetables (no fruit)

- Fruit (eaten, not juiced)

- Beet (stalks, leaves and root)

- Herbs for liver cleansing

- Chicory

- Astragalus

- Artemisia Capillaris (Wormwood)

- Turmeric (be sure to buy from a company that guarantees their turmeric is lead-free)

- Cilantro/Coriander

- Peppermint oil

- Artichoke

- Chinese salvia

- Chicory

- Dandelion

- Milk thistle/Silymarin

- Brown algae (ecklonia cava)

- Kudzu (pueraria lobata)

There are many other vitamins, minerals, enzymes, and herbs that have liver cleansing, building, and/or protective properties. To make a complete list would be impossible. The above list, however, should be more than adequate to draw from if you are interested in cleansing and supporting your liver.

Chapter Thirteen

What You Should Know About LDN & Its Benefits to Your Health

L DN Breaks all the rules.

In my long years of experience in the realm of healthcare, there has always been a divide between natural medicine and pharmacological medicine. A thing was either natural or it was pharmacological. One or the other, never both.

But there is one medicine that breaks this rule. It's known in the pharmaceutical realm as Naltrexone, and at regular doses of 50 to 200 mg, it is used to help opiate addicts and alcoholics break their addiction. In the natural realm of healing, however, it is called LDN (low-dose Naltrexone), and at extremely low doses of 4.5 mg or less, it is being used as a treatment in an impressive number of health conditions.

Does LDN work?

The short answer is yes. It absolutely works. A great deal of research has been done proving the effectiveness of low-dose Naltrexone, and more is currently in progress. Its value in the treatment of many health conditions is undisputed, and there is a long list of other conditions in which LDN therapy shows great promise.

The following is a statement taken from the LDN Research Trust website regarding LDN:

It reduces pain and fights inflammation. It is used to treat cancers, autoimmune diseases, chronic pain, and mental health issues, to name a few. Treatment is constantly evolving, with new conditions and methods of treatment being shared regularly.

The LDN Research Trust website is an excellent resource for anyone who wishes to know more about LDN. There you will find an extensive list of conditions that have been proven to respond to LDN as well as conditions in which LDN therapy shows promise. On the website, there is a plethora of information about how LDN works, how it's prescribed, and even a list of prescribers in different countries, broken down by states and/or cities in each country.

Change happens slowly in medicine.

So-called 'new advances' generally aren't new at all. In most cases, they have been around for 20 to 50 years before finally being embraced by the mainstream. LDN therapy is gradually gaining momentum, but despite the huge amount of research that has been done and the fact that numerous favorable articles have appeared in medical journals on the topic of LDN, only a small minority of doctors are prescribing it.

Because low-dose Naltrexone is an off-label use of the medication naltrexone, it cannot be purchased at a regular pharmacy. Doctors who prescribe LDN prescribe it via compounding pharmacies, where it is made into the form preferred by the prescribing doctor, the most popular (and convenient) being capsules. The doctor will generally start the patient on a very low dose, such as 1 mg or 1.5 mg, and gradually raise the dose over time increments of 4 days to 1 week until reaching the doctor's recommended maximum for that patient, usually 4.5 mg.

The traditional recommendation for taking LDN has been once a day at bedtime. The rationale for this has been that LDN triggers the release of endorphins and because the body generally releases endorphins at night, it is best to take it at bedtime. However, there are doctors who claim that patients who take LDN during the day are seeing the same benefits as those who take it at night. The research goes on.

Fortunately, LDN side effects are nothing scary, and if it is prescribed and taken correctly, side effects are fairly rare, mostly having to do with sleep and vivid dreams.

Conditions that respond to LDN therapy

As I previously mentioned, the LDN Research Trust website has a list of conditions in which LDN may be of benefit. I counted well over 300 conditions on this list, including many forms of cancer. If you struggle with any health condition, you may want to go on that website and see if yours is listed. You will probably be amazed at the incredibly wide range of effectiveness of LDN.

Below is a list of the main categories of health conditions that have been shown to benefit from LDN therapy. Each of the conditions listed below is a broad heading under which numerous other, more specific health conditions are listed.

Arthritis

Autoimmune disorders

Blood disorders

Cancers

Cardiac (heart) diseases

Chronic pain

Dermatologic (skin) diseases

Disorders of blood vessels

Disorders of the ears, nose, sinus, and throat

Disorders of the immune system

Endocrine diseases

Eye diseases

Gastrointestinal diseases

Infectious diseases

Kidney diseases

Liver disorders

Lung diseases

Neurologic conditions

Pediatric disorders (yes, children can take LDN too)

Psychological disorders

Sleep disorders

Women's disorders

And much more...

Why don't all doctors prescribe LDN?

After reading a list of the proven and possible healing effects of LDN, you will surely wonder how it could be that something so potentially valuable to the human race could be ignored by the bulk of the medical profession. How can they justify denying their patients the far-reaching benefits of such an amazing medicine? you might well ask, especially in view of the fact that for a large number of the conditions that LDN is being used for, medical science offers only drugs for symptomatic relief – and they are drugs that have numerous side effects.

The answer lies in human nature.

Doctors are humans, after all, and they tend to become set in their ways. Throughout human history, there have always been a few bold, large-minded, forward-thinking individuals who have formed the avant-garde in any new endeavor. The others hang back and wait until the groundwork is laid, the bridges built, and the road cleared before venturing out from their secure places or their lazy ignorance to try and claim a piece of the glory. It has always been that way in the medical world.

Give it time.

Meanwhile, there are online resources that can assist you in finding an LDN prescriber near you.

If you do find a doctor who is willing to write you a prescription for LDN, you may want to visit the LDN Research Trust website to make sure your prescriber is making the proper dosing recommendations. I have seen numerous cases in which a patient's doctor had prescribed LDN at too high a dosage, or the wrong dosing time, or made some other recommendation that would completely negate the potential benefits of the medication. LDN must be taken the right way, or don't bother taking it at all. And remember, with LDN, more is not better. If you are getting results from taking a single dose of LDN, taking two doses will NOT double your results. It will most likely stop them.

It's called low dose for a reason.

Chapter Fourteen

Autoimmune Disease

J ust maybe you don't just have to live with it.

Like all other degenerative diseases, autoimmune disease was formerly quite rare and is now disturbingly common and rapidly increasing in occurrence. The reasons for this are unquestionably the usual suspects: Our unhealthy food supply, our unhealthy lifestyle, and our unhealthy environment (including chemicals we use on, in, and around our bodies).

I have written extensively about these 'usual suspects' in other articles, so I won't go into them in great detail in this article. I will, however, reference other articles I have written that contain information of relevance to the subject of autoimmune disease.

I will also repeat the following statement which appears in a number of my other articles: In the natural realm of healing, it is recognized that the first task that needs to be performed when treating any patient is to eliminate the cause(s) of their disease.

Which begs the question: what is the cause (or causes) of autoimmune disease?

An article published in the medical journal Autoimmunity Reviews, on January 7, 2008, makes the following introductory statement:

"The etiology (cause) of autoimmune diseases is multifactorial: genetic, environmental, hormonal, and immunological factors are all considered important in their development. Nevertheless, the onset of at least 50% of autoimmune disorders has been attributed to "unknown trigger factors".

So, the causes of autoimmune diseases can be genetic, environmental, hormonal, or immunological . . . or unknown (at least half of the time).

An article in the Journal of the American Medical Association on June 19, 2018, states:

"Psychiatric reactions to life stressors are common in the general population and may result in immune dysfunction. Whether such reactions contribute to the risk of autoimmune disease remains unclear."

Psychiatric reactions to life stressors may be a cause of autoimmune disease.

But check this next one out...

A 2006 article in the medical journal Neuroimmunomodulation makes the following statement:

"Stress is now recognized as an important risk factor in the pathogenesis of autoimmune rheumatic diseases (i.e., rheumatoid arthritis)."

Stress!!

We all have stress. It's unavoidable. And it can cause health problems, including, apparently, autoimmune disease. However, psychiatric reactions to life stressors go beyond simple stress and take us into the realm of the mental health professional. We will leave them to do their work, and we will do ours.

I have often found, when dealing with patients who suffer from autoimmune disorders, that there has been a domino effect, beginning with a traumatic event (or a series of traumatic events) such as the death of a loved one, a divorce, or some other extremely stressful occurrence. In these cases, often the first domino to topple is the adrenals.

It's no secret that the adrenal glands, often referred to as our stress glands, can be adversely affected by stress and emotional trauma. When these all-important and very neglected glands begin to hypo-function, their output of important hormones, including testosterone, DHEA, cortisol, epinephrine (adrenaline), and others, can decrease. This can result in any number of health problems.

A note about adrenal hypo-function:

This is a controversial subject. The terms adrenal fatigue and adrenal exhaustion are not accepted medical terms. Adrenal insufficiency is the accepted medical diagnosis, and it is generally considered to be a condition of extreme hypofunction, even Addison's disease in which the adrenals fail to produce sufficient cortisol and aldosterone. This belief rules out the possibility of the adrenals producing insufficient amounts of other important adrenal hormones like testosterone and DHEA. I contend that any gland can function at a suboptimal level, which can affect the levels of any or all hormones produced by that gland. Hypo-function of a gland can be minimal or severe or to any degree in between. It happens to the thyroid, the pituitary, the pancreas, the ovaries, the parathyroid, and so forth. They can all hypofunction to a mild, moderate, or severe degree. It makes no sense to believe the adrenal glands are the exclusive exception. However, it gets a little more complicated; a better term than adrenal fatigue or adrenal exhaustion, and a more defining one, is hypothalamic-pituitary-adrenal axis dysregulation (which involves a constellation of symptoms).

When the adrenals are hypo-functioning, usually the next domino to fall is the thyroid. In clinical practice, I have found that people who have been diagnosed with hypothyroidism almost always, when asked, can correlate the onset of their symptoms with a time during or shortly after some traumatic or highly stressful life event.

Sound familiar? Yes. Four paragraphs ago I wrote about the same correlation between autoimmune disease and emotional trauma/stress. Interesting, don't you think?

The Next Domino

An article was published in March 2022 in the medical journal Diabetes Metabolic Journal titled Links between Thyroid Disorders and Glucose Homeostasis. In that article, the following statements appear:

"Thyroid disorders and diabetes mellitus often coexist and are closely related. Several studies have shown a higher prevalence of thyroid disorders in patients with diabetes mellitus and vice versa."

"TH (thyroid hormone) affects glucose homeostasis, and thyroid disorders and DM (diabetes mellitus) are associated with each other. Autoimmunity is an important element in the relationship between T1DM (type 1 diabetes mellitus) and AITD (autoimmune thyroid disease). Thyroid dysfunction, both hyperthyroidism and hypothyroidism, is associated with insulin resistance and T2DM."

So, Let's Connect the Dots:

1. Stress/emotional trauma can cause autoimmune disease:

2. Stress/emotional trauma can cause adrenal hypofunction

3. Adrenal hypofunction can result in thyroid hypofunction

4. Thyroid disorders and autoimmune disease are "closely related" to insulin resistance and type 1 and type 2 diabetes.

Doesn't it seem obvious that to simply treat the particular gland that is hypo-functioning is to ignore the overall picture? If the forest is dying, treating the symptoms of the tree that is directly in front of you will accomplish very little.

Other causes of autoimmune disease

I'll repeat the statement from the medical journal Autoimmunity Reviews, January 7, 2008, referenced at the beginning of this article:

"The etiology (cause) of autoimmune diseases is multifactorial: genetic, environmental, hormonal, and immunological factors are all considered important in their development."

In other words, in addition to stress/emotional trauma, there can be other causes of autoimmune disease. And, in the natural realm of healing, we believe in dealing with the causes!

There's the challenge. How can you know what is causing the autoimmune condition in a particular person? Please read on. I think I can help you with that conundrum. (hint: start by eliminating the usual suspects)

Autoimmune disease can present in many different ways and can affect any part of the body. I went to a website called Autoimmune Registry. On this website, they have a list of autoimmune diseases listed in alphabetical order. I counted 169 diseases on that list.

We don't really understand why different people have different areas of the body that are being attacked by their own immune system, and this whole scenario may seem overwhelming to the health professional who is trying to help someone who is suffering from an autoimmune disorder.

It doesn't have to be overwhelming if you remember the following rules:

1. Treat the patient, not the disease (or the symptoms of the disease).

2. The body is perfectly able to heal itself if given the right help.

3. The first job is to remove the cause(s) or potential cause(s) of the disease. In most instances, that involves cleansing.

4. The number one most important subject regarding human health is nutrition. Destructive nutritional factors cause disease, and healthful nutritional factors enable the body to heal itself.

5. Heal the liver and heal the gut. Repeat that statement 10 times and burn it into your memory.

6. Never forget that only natural things are compatible with our natural organisms. (see my article on the law of compatibility)

If you understand the above rules, if you truly own them, the task of assisting the body to heal and normalize its immune system becomes not so overwhelming after all. In fact, the information you need is probably all right here on this website in different articles on various subjects. In fact, with the inclusion of the article you are now reading, I believe you will find a blueprint for health (including immune health). Below is a list of the titles of the articles I believe to be pertinent to the subject of autoimmune disease:

- What you need to know about LDN. This article deals with a natural/prescription medicine that I believe to be a must in dealing with a person who suffers from any form of autoimmune disorder.

- Leaky Gut. You may have it. A leaky gut can cause autoimmune disease, as well as a host of other health disorders.

- Chronic inflammation. This article deals with leaky gut, which can also cause autoimmune disorders.

- Insulin resistance. This issue definitely needs to be corrected in cases of autoimmune disorders.

- The much-ignored tragedy of Candidiasis. Discusses causes, symptoms, and treatment of systemic candidiasis—another cause of autoimmune diseases.

- Breaking your sugar addiction. Sugar has been implicated in almost every degenerative disease known to man, including autoimmune disease.

- Toxic sweeteners. Need I say more?

- PCOS. Related to insulin resistance.

- How to lose weight and keep it off. This article addresses leptin resistance and all the issues it can cause, including autoimmune disorders; it also addresses how to correct leptin resistance.

- The life-saving benefits of vitamin K. This article is a must-read.

- Healthy liver, healthy life. Proper liver function is essential for general health and immune health.

- Dealing with Depression and Anxiety. Because of the established emotional connection between emotional factors and autoimmune disease, the information in this article may play a crucial role in helping autoimmune victims.

The above articles all dovetail perfectly with each other and form a net of information that can create an understanding of the different factors that individually or in combination, are causes of autoimmune disease. Each article also provides a list of natural substances that have been scientifically shown to benefit patients, along with dosages.

Whether you are a health professional or an individual seeking scientific answers to your autoimmune health condition, I'm certain the heavily researched information provided in these articles will be of great value to you. As a subscriber to this newsletter, you already have access to them.

One last note on some recent research regarding autoimmune disorders:

Research has indicated that drinking baking soda in water may be an effective treatment in cases of rheumatoid arthritis and other autoimmune disorders.

An article in Medical News Today states: "A daily dose of baking soda may help reduce the destructive inflammation of autoimmune diseases like rheumatoid arthritis, scientists say. They have some of the first evidence of how the cheap, over-the-counter antacid can encourage our spleen to promote instead an anti-inflammatory environment that could be therapeutic in the face of inflammatory disease, Medical College of Georgia scientists report in the Journal of Immunology."

It appears that baking soda shifts the balance of immune cells, decreasing the number of inflammatory immune cells while elevating the number of anti-inflammatory cells.

It is still under investigation, but it seems that this is yet another potential benefit of that versatile and health-promoting substance, sodium bicarbonate, (baking soda).

Below is a list of some of the usual suspects:

- Sugar and chemical sweeteners.

- Vegetable oils (seed oils).

- Harmful beverages (you know what they are. Just drink pure water)

- MSG (monosodium glutamate) Like many criminals, this one goes by many aliases.

- GMO (genetically modified) foods.

- Gluten

- Commercial dairy products (butter is fine; butter substitutes are not)

- Chemicals in foods and water: (pesticides, caffeine, fluoride, Teflon. . . well, it's a long list).

- Antibiotics or anything else that harms our biome (beneficial bacteria)

- Tobacco, alcohol, and vaping (but you already knew that).

- Chemicals in personal products: Hair color, antiperspirants, some shampoos, and cosmetics (it's another long list)

As I said, this is only a partial list.

The point is our bodies are natural, and only natural things are compatible with them. I call it the law of compatibility.

Cortisol Dysregulation: Chances Are You Have It – Your Health May Be at Risk

It's a stressful world, sometimes even a scary one. Much is often expected of us, and sometimes it's hard to perform all the tasks and accomplish all the things that are required of us. In short, life can get overwhelming.

And cortisol can become dysregulated.

Cortisol is a steroid hormone produced by the adrenal glands and adipose (fatty) tissue. It is the body's primary stress hormone, acting on different parts of the brain to control different emotions.

Below is a list of some of the functions of cortisol in the body:

- Has a huge impact on mood. It also affects motivation and fear.

- Controls blood pressure

- Suppresses inflammation

- Prevents low blood sugar

- Boosts energy during stressful times

- Manages metabolism of proteins, fats, and carbs

- Controls sleep/wake cycle

Having an occasional elevation of cortisol is not a problem. It's chronic cortisol dysregulation that causes so many health problems—some of them very serious.

The following is a list of some of the problems that can be caused by cortisol dysregulation:

- Facial weight gain (moon face)

- Abdominal weight gain (central obesity/belly fat)

- Fatty deposits around the shoulder blades

- Increased appetite with a preference for high glycemic, high caloric foods

- Sugar cravings

- All the components of metabolic syndrome

- Cardiovascular disease

- Increased blood pressure

- Increased blood sugar

- Type 2 diabetes

- Low sex drive

- Depression

- Anxiety

- Insomnia

- Low energy

- Reduction of growth hormone production

- Inflammation

- Thinning hair on the scalp

- Increased body hair, primarily in women

- Weakened muscles in thighs and upper arms

- Purple abdominal stretch marks

- Weakening of bones

- Many more

- Loss of muscle and bone mass

Because cortisol is catabolic (as opposed to anabolic), if you are trying to build muscle, elevated cortisol will fight against you It can actually reduce muscle mass, as well as bone mass. At the same time, fat will accumulate, especially on your belly and face.

There can be a definite overlap between symptoms of cortisol dysregulation and symptoms of hypothyroidism and menopause. Sorting this all out can be challenging because cortisol dysregulation can depress thyroid function and aggravate menopausal symptoms. It can also cause blood sugar dysregulation, which can cause multiple symptoms and even result in type 2 diabetes.

As a result, cortisol dysregulation is often misdiagnosed as something else and is left completely untreated.

Testing Cortisol Levels

Some health professionals will use blood tests to check their patient's cortisol levels.

Continue reading, and I will explain why the results of a single blood draw are diagnostically useless and why blood testing is not the best way to check cortisol levels.

Cortisol is released in a pulsatile manner. Different amounts of it are released into the blood at various times during the day. Blood levels of cortisol can fluctuate drastically from morning to night. Under normal circumstances, cortisol levels go down at night so we can sleep and begin to rise in the early morning so we can wake up and be alert when we start our day.

In other words, sometimes blood cortisol levels are supposed to be at a low level and sometimes they are supposed to be higher.

Another thing to consider is that it is estimated that blood cortisol levels can go up as much as nine hundred percent during a stressful event.

Doing a blood draw to check the level of cortisol will only give a snapshot of where cortisol is at that exact moment.

Furthermore, blood tests for the steroid hormones (of which cortisol is one) are not able to isolate the free portion of the hormone (which is the biologically active portion) from the protein-bound portion (which is not fully biologically active). The free portion of a hormone is estimated to be only between one and ten percent of the total amount of that hormone in the blood at any given time.

There is a Better Test for Cortisol Levels

In my opinion, saliva testing is a far more accurate way to test cortisol levels. Here's why:

1. Saliva tests detect the level of the free, biologically active portion of the cortisol in the body.

2. The patient has the test kit at home with several sample vials and is able to take samples at intervals throughout a twenty-four hour period, thus providing information regarding the fluctuations of cortisol, as well as an average. This is truly useful information as compared to a blood draw which is only a snapshot.

3. No needles are involved in saliva testing, thus eliminating the possibility of a surge of cortisol caused by fear of the needle and/or the stress of 'white coat syndrome.' Sometimes just driving to a clinic and being in that environment can cause cortisol to go up.

4. Saliva testing is highly accurate.

(As an aside, the above information on testing applies to all the steroid hormones—the estrogens, progesterone, testosterone, DHEA, etc.)

Hair Analysis Hormone Testing

Hair analysis is another form of testing that can be very helpful, giving a longer-term average of cortisol levels than either blood, saliva, or urine testing.

Urine Hormone Testing

Urine testing is another method of testing cortisol levels. It is a good adjunct to saliva tests, as it tests the metabolites of the hormone which is information that is valued by many clinicians. However, I personally do not feel that urine tests can replace saliva tests for cortisol and sex steroids.

Cortisol and Menopause

It's a well-known fact that cortisol interacts with other hormones. Studies have shown that cortisol dysregulation may cause early menopause and that regulating cortisol levels may help ameliorate menopausal symptoms.

Cortisol and the Thyroid

A study published in the medical science journal Cureus on Dec. 15, 2023, makes the following statement:

"The study's results emphasize the complex interaction between cortisol and thyroid function, suggesting a direct relationship between serum cortisol and TSH levels in hypothyroidism. Patients with severe hypothyroidism exhibited elevated cortisol concentrations . . . "

Other studies have shown a connection between elevated cortisol levels and low thyroid function (hypothyroidism). It is clear that elevated cortisol levels can put the thyroid into a state of decreased activity.

Cortisol and Obesity

In an article published in the medical journal Obesity (Siver Spring) in April 2018, the authors make the following statement: ". . . higher cortisol, insulin, and chronic stress were each predictive of

greater future weight gain."

Keeping in mind that excess cortisol can cause all the health problems that are the components of metabolic syndrome, it is interesting to note that those same health conditions can cause an increase in cortisol production. Does that sound like a vicious cycle to you?

Cortisol and Leptin

I have written about leptin in other articles, particularly those concerning weight loss. Leptin levels and leptin resistance have a huge impact on weight control and obesity in humans.

How leptin functions in the body is extremely complex, and we are not even close to fully understanding it. We do know, however, that leptin is primarily produced in white adipose tissue (fat) and that it communicates with the brain, telling the brain when the body has adequate fuel. The brain then does two things: It tells the body to stop eating (decreased appetite), and it stimulates the metabolism so more calories will be burned. But, when there is a state of leptin resistance, the brain does not receive the message, and it thinks the body is starving. It thinks you need more food, so it lowers the metabolic rate and stimulates the appetite. Now, you are consuming more calories and burning fewer. This results in stored fuel in the form of fat deposits on the body, and a very frustrated person. Sound familiar?

Glucocorticoids (cortisol is one of them) stimulate the release of leptin from fatty tissue, while at the same time reducing leptin sensitivity in the brain. This can result in leptin resistance. I suspect this apparent contradiction is related to the amounts of glucocorticoids present in the blood. It may simply come down to what we already know: too much cortisol causes too many problems.

Cortisol and Leaky Gut

High cortisol levels can trigger leaky gut syndrome, causing systemic inflammation, another causative factor for leptin resistance and many other health problems.

Cortisol dysregulation is just another example of how the modern diet and lifestyle are causing an epidemic of obesity and chronic disease.

Chapter Sixteen

Can Blood Pressure Be Controlled Without a Prescription? What Is the Science?

We all know that high blood pressure can be dangerous. But so can blood pressure medications; they have a lot of side effects, some of them very undesirable.

It would seem a safe assumption that no health professional would be unhappy if any of their patients were to be able to control their blood pressure using natural means thus eliminating the need for blood pressure medications.

But can blood pressure really be controlled without prescription medications?

There are many research studies reported on PubMed that claim it can. Here are some excerpts from a few of them:

Note: I have highlighted certain relevant sections of these research reports.

Phytotherapy of Hypertension: An Updated Overview

Mohammed Ajebli 1, Mohamed Eddouks 1

PMID: 31880255

Recent evidence from clinical trials suggests that a wide variety of herbal preparations and plant extracts or natural isolated compounds have a favorable therapeutic impact on blood flow . . .Hence, based on the findings of the present review, medicinal plant derivatives could be used as preventive and curative agents in the case of cardiovascular disorders, particularly hypertension, and could play a promoting function in the discovery of new antihypertensive agents.

Mechanisms underlying the antihypertensive effects of garlic bio-actives

Reem Shouk 1, Aya Abdou 2, Kalidas Shetty 3, Dipayan Sarkar 3, Ali H Eid 4

PMID: 24461311

This review suggests that garlic and garlic-derived bio-actives have significant medicinal properties with the potential for ameliorating hypertension and associated morbidity.

Dietary supplements in the management of hypertension and diabetes - a review

Anthony Jide Afolayan 1, Olubunmi Abosede Wintola

PMID: 25371590

Result and discussion: This review chronicled the therapeutic values of vitamins, minerals, amino acids, fruits, vegetables, herbs, and other botanicals used as dietary supplements. Results show that these supplements provided better and safer substitutes for toxic and expensive conventional drugs. Generally, dietary supplements are free from major side effects, readily available, and affordable. It is envisaged that the use of dietary supplements will promote good health and improve the status of hypertensive and diabetic patients.

Conclusion: Medical doctors are therefore encouraged to incorporate dietary supplements into the regimen employed for hypertension and diabetes management.

The Potential of Natural Products in the Management of Cardiovascular Disease

Harshita Singhai 1, Sunny Rathee 1, Sanjay K Jain 1, Umesh Kumar Patil 1

PMID: 38477208

Conventional treatments for CVDs (cardiovascular diseases) are often quite expensive and also have several side effects.

This potentiates the use of medicinal plants, which are still a viable alternative therapy for a number of diseases, including CVD (cardiovascular disease). Natural products' cardio-protective effects result from their anti-oxidative, anti-hypercholesterolemia, anti-ischemic, and platelet aggregation-inhibiting properties.

On PubMed, there are many thousands of articles similar to the above, discussing the healing properties of natural substances for a myriad of health conditions, including high blood pressure.

Below, I will provide a list of some of those natural healing agents, but first a list of the common causes of hypertension.

Common causes of hypertension:

- Sugar (this includes high fructose corn syrup and agave)

- Seed (vegetable) oils

- Lack of exercise

- Obesity (all 3 of the above factors are common causes of obesity)

- Tobacco

- Alcohol

- Some medications, such as pain relievers, birth control pills, cold and cough preparations, and other prescription drugs

- Illegal drugs

- Sleep apnea

- Hypercortisolism (I have written about this problem, which is extremely common, rarely diagnosed, and almost always untreated)

These are some natural medicines that have been proven scientifically to lower blood pressure.

The dosages listed below are those commonly used.

- Garlic: No dosage has been established.

- Magnesium taurate: 500 to 1,000 mg daily.

- Vitamin D3: 5,000 iu daily

- Vitamin K2. (K2,7, (MK7)) 500 mcg daily

- Bergamot: 500-1500 mg daily

- L-Arginine: 5 or 6 thousand mg per day in divided doses.

- Vitamin C: I recommend Kakadu plum powder (on Amazon)

- Beetroot juice. Fresh juiced, organic.

- CoQ10: 200 mg daily

- Controlled release melatonin: 2.5 mg 1 hour before bedtime.

- Lycopene: 8 to 30 mg daily

- Rhodiola: 100 mg daily to begin with, building up to 200 mg twice daily.

- Reducing calcium intake can also help to lower blood pressure in some cases

- Potassium: Varies per need

Exercise is important

Controlling cortisol levels is essential

Hypertension is one of the many health conditions in which science-based non-pharmacological medicine can be highly beneficial.

Chapter Seventeen

There's Hope for Fibromyalgia Sufferers – It's Time to Learn More

Fibromyalgia is real; anyone who has it can attest to that fact. The pain is real, the malaise is real, and the mental and emotional aspects of it are real as well.

But fibromyalgia is not a disease; it's not a diagnosis; it's a collection of symptoms. The name itself is a description of the symptoms. Fibro refers to the fibrous tissues, myo means muscle, and algia means pain. So, the term fibromyalgia literally means pain in the muscles and fibrous tissues of the body.

Pain is not a diagnosis; it's a symptom.

Conventional medical providers treat the symptoms of fibromyalgia with drugs.

A report published in April 2021 in the International Journal of Molecular Science makes the following statement regarding fibromyalgia:

"Unfortunately, the conventional medical therapies that target this pathology produce limited benefits. They remain largely pharmacological in nature and tend to treat the symptomatic aspects . . . The statistics, however, highlight the fact that 90% of people with fibromyalgia also turn to complementary medicine to manage their symptoms."

If you have Fibromyalgia and your health professional is merely treating your symptoms with drugs, you may want to look elsewhere for answers. Read on, and you may find some.

In the natural realm of healing, we deal with the causes of disease and human suffering. Everything has a cause, and Fibromyalgia is no exception. The cause or causes may differ from patient to patient. Multiple factors can produce the symptoms known as Fibromyalgia, and each of these factors must be dealt with because they can all create other diseases as well—some of them very serious.

The good news is, if you correct the cause(s) of your Fibromyalgia symptoms, you will be doing great benefit to your health in countless other ways.

What causes Fibromyalgia?

Medical professionals will generally tell the patient that the causes are unknown and will proceed to treat the symptoms with drugs. I recently read on a website the statement, "Fibromyalgia has no cure."

Please do not accept that!

Just because there is no drug to cure it doesn't mean there is no cure. And just because conventional medical providers do not know the causes, does not mean they are not known.

According to the information posted on the website of Mayo Clinic, the following are possible causes of Fibromyalgia:

- Genetics

- Infections

- Physical or emotional events

....Yawn......same old information.

Here's my opinion on that:

Genetics: We can't change our genetics, but there's no solid connection between fibromyalgia and genetics other than the fact that it is more common in some families than others. Moreover, a genetic predisposition is just that: a predisposition. It doesn't mean fibro is unavoidable in your case, nor does it mean you can't do anything about it if you have it.

Infections: Yes, infections; viral, bacterial, fungal, and even parasitic, can cause fibromyalgia symptoms. You may think the answer to that would be antibiotics.

Think again.

Antibiotics can cause many health problems. They can even cause damage that can lead to fibromyalgia. They can also cause microorganisms to become antibiotic-resistant. Antibiotic-resistant bacteria are often referred to as superbugs. These superbugs are dangerous. They kill many people every year.

In fibromyalgia cases, I do not believe antibiotics are the answer. I believe they will only add to your problems.

There are bacterial and viral infections that do not show up on routine blood tests, so the fact that blood tests show no infection doesn't mean you have no infection.

So, what's the answer?

Physical or emotional events: That's pretty vague. I agree that trauma—physical or emotional—can cause fibromyalgia symptoms, but the question is, how does it do that?

It is a well-known fact that stress (physical or emotional) can affect what is known as the HPA (hypothalamic-pituitary-adrenal) axis. This can result in, among other things, hypofunction of the adrenal glands, (sometimes referred to as adrenal fatigue, adrenal insufficiency, or adrenal exhaustion).

One of the hormones produced by the adrenal glands is cortisol, which performs many functions, one of which is to control inflammation in the body.

A report published in Sept 2010 in the International Journal of Behavioral Medicine, with the title: Fibromyalgia syndrome is associated with hypocortisolism, states the following:

"Patients with FMS (fibromyalgia syndrome) had significantly lower cortisol levels during the day, most pronounced in the morning . . . As expected, FMS patients reported more pain, stress, sleeping problems, anxiety, and depression. Conclusion: The results lend support to the hypothesis of a dysfunction in the hypothalamus-pituitary-adrenal axis in FMS patients, with generally lower cortisol values, most pronounced upon awakening."

Other potential causes of Fibromyalgia syndrome

Metal Toxicity

A 2013 article in the journal Neuro Endocrinology Letters entitled,

Metal-induced inflammation triggers fibromyalgia in metal-allergic patients, makes the following statement:

"Metal allergy is frequent in FM (fibromyalgia) patients. The reduction of metal exposure resulted in improved health in the majority of metal-sensitized patients. This suggests that metal-induced inflammation might be an important risk factor in a subset of patients with FM."

One thing is very clear: there are different causes of fibromyalgia syndrome, but there is

strong evidence that one of them is metal toxicity. In this study, mercury from "dental restorations" (probably mercury amalgam fillings), nickel, cadmium, and lead, were the ones that were most commonly reacted to.

Many functional medicine clinics begin their treatment regimens by recommending the patient have any and all mercury removed from their mouth.

Dysbiosis and Leaky Gut

It is my opinion that the majority of cases of fibromyalgia syndrome will respond extremely well to the right program dealing with intestinal dysbiosis and intestinal hyperpermeability (aka leaky gut).

Hippocrates said, "All disease begins in the gut."

With just a few exceptions, I believe this to be one of the great truths. Generally speaking, in our modern society, not only do we not take effective measures to heal the gut and maintain gut health, but almost everything we do and many things we consume (including our medications) damage the gut biome.

The intestinal biome (beneficial bacteria) is becoming increasingly understood and is now considered to be another organ, and it constitutes over 80% of our immune system. Damage to your biome equals damage to your health.

Below are some common causes of destruction of the intestinal biome:

Some medications, such as antibiotics, corticosteroids, birth control pills, and others. (remember, many commercial dairy, fish, and meat products contain antibiotics that were administered to the animal, bird, or fish during its life. (Another reason to eat organic)

- Chlorinated water

- Junk foods with all their chemicals and lack of nutrients

- Failure to eat the proper foods that nourish and replenish the beneficial bacteria

- Alcohol

- Tobacco

- Pesticides and chemicals in foods

- Artificial sweeteners (maybe)

- Stress

- Candida Albicans (See my article on Candidiasis)

- Poor sleep habits

- Insufficient exercise

- Chronic constipation

In other words; the modern diet and lifestyle.

A few of the diseases that have been associated with dysbiosis (damaged intestinal microbiota) are:

- Fibromyalgia

- Chronic fatigue syndrome

- Colitis

- Irritable bowel disease

- Other gastrointestinal inflammatory diseases

- Autoimmune diseases

- Intestinal hyperpermeability (leaky gut)

- SIBO (small intestine bacterial overgrowth)

- Gynecological disorders (the gut biome has a great impact on the vaginal biome)

- Systemic candidiasis

- Hormonal issues (the gut biome is considered to be a full-fledged endocrine organ)

- Metabolic conditions (like diabetes)

- Respiratory diseases

- Neurological conditions

- Neurological conditions

- Cardiovascular conditions

Much More

A recent article in the scientific journal Frontiers in Cellular and Infection Microbiology states the following: Recent studies suggest a potential connection between certain gut bacteria and female reproductive tract disorders, such as bacterial vaginosis (BV), cervical and endometrial cancer, polycystic ovary syndrome (PCOS), post-menopausal syndrome, endometriosis, endometritis, and uterine fibroids (UFs)

It's very clear that the health (or disease) of the gut microbiome affects every part of the body.

So, what can be done about Dysbiosis and Leaky Gut Syndrome?

For starters, avoid the things on the list below:

Healing the gut requires a multifaceted approach, the obvious first step of which is to avoid the things that caused the problem to begin with. See a partial list of those things, below.

- Sugar (including high fructose corn syrup and agave)

- Pasteurized dairy products. (butter is healthy. Avoid butter substitutes)

- Gluten

- Chlorinated water.

- Seed oils (vegetable oils)

- Junk foods with all their chemicals and lack of nutrients

- Low fiber diet

- Failure to eat the proper foods that nourish and replenish the beneficial bacteria.

- Alcohol

- Tobacco

- Pesticides and chemicals in foods

- Artificial sweeteners (maybe)

- Harmful beverages like soda, energy drinks, sports drinks, and others. These harm the health in numerous ways.

Certain medications cause dysbiosis by killing the microbiota. Antibiotics, for example, don't know when to stop killing. They kill the good bacteria along with the bad. However, If you are taking a prescribed medication, you should consult a qualified healthcare professional before stopping. Don't try to do it alone.

Re-establish the intestinal biome.

Once the individual has eliminated the causative factors, they need to begin re-establishing the intestinal biome. Below are some recommendations for accomplishing that.

Butyrate

Nothing is more important than butyrate for gut health and for the health of the beneficial bacteria in the gut. In a normal gut or in a diseased gut, butyrate is essential. It is also essential in dealing with leaky gut syndrome. Below is a list of butyrate-producing foods. The term butyrate-producing foods means they are foods that feed the bacteria in the gut that produce butyrate.

- Vegetable fiber. Eat lots of fresh, raw, organic vegetables.

- Honey (MUST BE raw, organic, unprocessed).

- Sweet potato

- Zucchini

- Cruciferous vegetables

- Purple kale.

- Purple cabbage.

- Eggplant.

- Radish.

- Green banana (organic) (must be VERY GREEN), or you can buy green banana powder as a supplement.

- Probiotics, prebiotics, and fermented foods. These are essential for replenishing the intestinal biome. Many people think they can simply eat some yogurt and it will do the job. It won't.

Kill candida

If there is a problem with candidiasis, the candida needs to be taken under control. This requires specialized knowledge due to the biofilms the candida organism constructs to protect itself. Below, you will find information on how to eliminate candida and its biofilms.

Avoid constipation!

Constipation is much more than just a minor annoyance; it is potentially very harmful to the health and very damaging to the colon and the intestinal microbiota. Magnesium citrate and magnesium oxide are great natural laxatives.

Detoxify and heal the colon.

A few of the things that can help with colon detox and regeneration are:

Drinking a lot of purified water.

Drinking 2 large glasses of warm (approximately body temperature), purified water first thing in the morning on an empty stomach. Then, if possible, don't eat anything for ½ hour or more. This is a powerful healing remedy for the colon, the rest of the G.I. tract, the liver, and the kidneys. The water should be warmed on the stove, not in a microwave. Do not drink tap water.

Coconut charcoal. 1 or 2 capsules 3 times daily. This will adsorb many of the impurities in the intestinal tract and keep them from entering the blood.

Psyllium fiber. (Pronounced silly um) 2 to 4 tablespoons in a glass of water at bedtime.

Juicing fresh, raw, organic vegetables (not fruit)

Fermented foods. This is crucial!

L-Glutamine. This is an amino acid that is very beneficial to the colon. 5,000 - 10,000 mg daily is a common dosage.

Aloe vera

Slippery elm

Coconut oil

Butyrate. I mention butyrate again because it is so important. Remember, the key is not to eat butyrate-containing foods but to eat foods that feed the bacteria in the gut that produce butyrate. A list of those is provided above.

Herbs

There are a number of herbs that are beneficial in colon cleansing. Below is a partial list.

- Aloe vera

- Ginger

- Turmeric (use fresh turmeric root, or make sure your product is lead-free)

- Dandelion root

- Licorice root

- Fennel

- Mint

I've covered A LOT in the first part of this article. Don't miss part two which will be available next week. Next week you will learn more about living with the effects of Fibromyalgia.

There's Hope for Fibromyalgia Sufferers - It's Time to Learn More - Part Two

Candidiasis

How to effectively deal with candidiasis.

There are as many approaches to this problem as there are opinions. And for every opinion, there are a hundred natural candida cleanses, candida clears, candida fighters, killers, and what-have-yous sold in health food stores and online. Obviously, I haven't seen them all in action, but the ones I've seen haven't impressed me.

Most of them have some good ingredients, but they are inadequate. They don't address all the many complex aspects of dysbiosis and candidiasis.

I don't claim to have all the answers, I don't believe anyone does, nor could anyone possibly scrutinize all the mountains of scientific literature on this subject, but, if you suffer from this problem I am confident I can give you some information that will help.

Candidiasis is fixable, but it requires a multipronged approach. The dysbiosis has to be addressed, the biofilms have to be eliminated, the candida organisms have to be killed, and successive generations of fungi hatched from the eggs left by the previous generation also have to be killed off, each generation becoming less numerous than the last; the body has to be cleansed, the intestinal hyperpermeability (leaky gut) has to be corrected, and the immune system has to be strengthened. Additionally, the individual has to change the habits that have created the problem and allow it to grow and continue.

It's a complex problem, and it requires a complex solution. Please continue reading.

Killing Candida

To eradicate candida, you must destroy its strongholds. Its biofilms.

The following is a list of natural substances that have been shown in scientific studies to eliminate biofilms and/or kill candida albicans. (Please understand that everyone has different needs, so the dosages in the lists below are guidelines only). I have divided the list into two categories: the substances that break down biofilms and also kill candida organisms, and those that kill candida, but may not affect the biofilms.

Natural antifungals have been shown scientifically to also eradicate biofilms:

**Enzymes. My preferred product for this purpose is, again, Flavenzyme from . (mentioned above) Dosage: 7 tablets first thing in the morning on an empty stomach, with 16 oz of purified water. Don't eat anything for 1½ to 2 hours, but continue drinking water every ½ hour until you eat. Do the same in the afternoon or evening if you can arrange to have an empty stomach.

**Xylitol - A natural, healthy sugar. (and, yes, diabetics can take it.)

Eucalyptus oil - ½ ml to 2 ml daily.

*NAC (N acetyl Cysteine) - 200 to 600 mg 3 times daily.

Colloidal silver - I prefer ionic silver (ACS 200 from Results RNA)

**Coconut oil (virgin, organic) -1 tablespoonful 3 times daily.

**Citrus Pectin - 10-20 grams daily

*Berberine - 500 mg 2 or 3 times daily.

EGCG - Start with 200 mg 2 times daily, build up over 1 month to 400 mg 2 times daily.

*Oregano oil - (Wld, Mediterranean) 1 drop in water 3 times daily. Build up to 2 drops 3 times daily.

*Piperine - 5 mg 3 times daily.

*Undecylenic acid - 250 mg 3 times daily.

Grapefruit seed extract - 10-12 drops in water 2 or 3 times daily.

Natural antifungals that kill candida but may not break down biofilms:

*Food-grade diatomaceous earth - 1 tsp one time daily, build up over 10 days to 1 tsp 2 times daily in water. Do not inhale. Must be food grade!

*Olive leaf extract - 500 mg 2 times daily

**Prebiotics

**Probiotics

**Fermented foods (essential)

I would not recommend trying to take everything on the above lists at once. I have placed a star next to the ones I have chosen as the primary ones. They are all excellent. The non-starred ones are also good but are optional. You may even want to alternate, taking the single-starred ones one week and the non-starred ones the next. The ones with 2 stars should be taken regardless of what else is taken.

The Candida Diet

An important aspect of killing candida involves starving the fungal organisms.

For in-depth nutritional recommendations, I recommend the website Their candida diet is healthy, and it will keep the candida from having any food source. They even have an e-book with candida-friendly recipes.

How to minimize die-off (Herxheimer) reaction.

Before you begin a candida program, be prepared for the inevitable die-off reaction. It usually lasts from 3 days to a week and can be minimized by the following:

Drink a lot of purified water

Coconut charcoal - 1 or 2 capsules 3 times daily. As previously stated, this will adsorb many of the impurities in the intestinal tract that are created by the die-off of the candida, and keep them from entering the blood.

Enzymes - My preferred product for this purpose is Flavenzyme from . Dosage: 7 tablets first thing in the morning on an empty stomach with 16 oz of purified water. Don't eat anything for 1½ to 2 hours, but continue drinking water every ½ hour until you eat. Do the same in the afternoon or evening if you can arrange to have an empty stomach. Taken this way, the enzymes will be very beneficial in cleansing the blood and minimizing Herxheimer reaction. The enzymes will also play a crucial role in breaking down the biofilms that protect the candida organisms.

Hormones and Fibromyalgia

There appears to be a strong hormonal component in fibromyalgia syndrome. One study of fibromyalgia patients found that when progesterone was low and cortisol was high, the patients experienced more pain.

I won't dwell on this issue here. I refer you to my articles on bioidentical hormones, saliva testing, and cortisol.

Lyme Disease and Fibromyalgia

This is a subject about which much has been written, owing to the fact that the symptoms of Lyme disease closely resemble those of fibromyalgia. Some research has shown that Lyme disease may trigger fibromyalgia; however, antibiotic therapy for Lyme disease does not seem to impact fibromyalgia symptoms.

Nutritional Supplements for Fibromyalgia

It appears that in fibromyalgia, the mitochondria (energy-producing organelles) in the cells are functioning at a sub-normal level, producing less energy. This is undoubtedly the reason why chronic fatigue syndrome is a frequent companion to fibromyalgia syndrome.

Therefore, an important aspect of a natural approach to this problem is to re-energize the mitochondria. Below, is a list of supplements that have been shown to be useful in supporting the mitochondria.

- D-Ribose

- Magnesium Glycinate

- Gynostemma

- Cordyceps

- CoQ10

- NADH

A research report in the scientific journal Antioxidants & Redox Signaling, 2015 Mar 10, bearing the title, Does Oral Coenzyme Q10 Plus NADH Supplementation Improve Fatigue and Biochemical Parameters in Chronic Fatigue Syndrome? makes the following statement:

"Emerging data suggest that CoQ10 and NADH deficiencies have been described in patients with chronic fatigue syndrome (CFS) and fibromyalgia (FMS). Both CoQ10 and NADH play a critical role in mitochondrial ATP production and cellular metabolism homeostasis.

It has been suggested that the combinations of natural antioxidant supplements can reduce significantly the fatigue and even naturally restore mitochondrial function in long-term CFS patients with intractable fatigue. Preliminary data have shown a remarkable clinical improvement after initiating oral NADH or CoQ10 supplementation in patients with CFS and FMS."

Low dose Naltrexone

I have discussed low-dose Naltrexone (LDN) in depth in another article, but I feel strongly that it needs to be mentioned briefly here. LDN is an off-label use of the drug Naltrexone. LDN has been shown to be beneficial in numerous diseases, including fibromyalgia and chronic fatigue syndrome. I am not recommending it, I'm only recommending that you learn about and discuss it with your healthcare provider if it interests you.

LDN is sold by prescription, and many medical providers are still not well informed on how to prescribe it and what its benefits are; I recommend that anyone who suffers from fibromyalgia read my article on the subject and go to the website to learn more about this amazing and very safe medicine.

Other supplements that are often used in Fibromyalgia cases

- Iodine (very important)

- Fish oil

- Vitamin D3 and vitamin K2 (MK7) (Important! Before taking, read my article on vitamin K2)

- Ashwagandha

- Turmeric

- Camu powder or Kakadu plum powder

- Rhodiola

- A trace mineral supplement (from the sea or from the Great Salt Lake)

The following is a list of supplements that have been used for the pain of Fibromyalgia

- Quercetin

- Myrrh

- St John's wort

- Choline

The following is a list of things that should be avoided by fibromyalgia sufferers (and everyone else)

- Gluten

- Sugar

- Caffeine

- Tobacco

- MSG (monosodium glutamate)

- Alcohol

- Artificial sweeteners

- Commercial dairy products (butter is OK, butter substitutes are not)

- Vegetable oils (seed oils)

- Trans fats

- Dehydration (drink a lot of water)

- Constipation (magnesium oxide powder can help)

- GMO foods

In summary, I do not believe the causes of fibromyalgia/chronic fatigue syndrome are unknown, nor do I believe there is no cure. And I speak from experience.

About the author

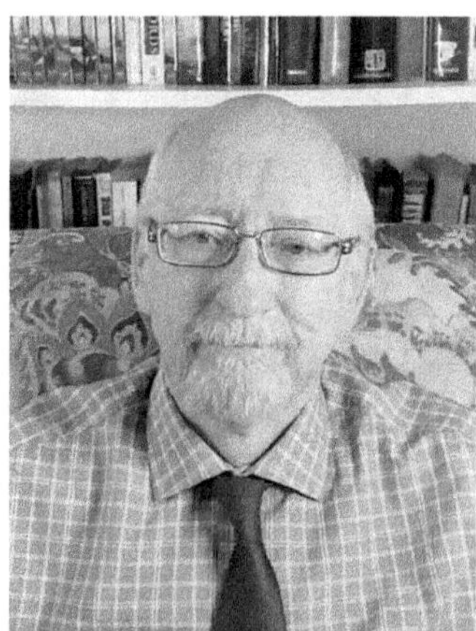

Dr. C.M. Curtis

For over four decades, Dr. C.M. Curtis has been a pioneering voice in health and wellness, bridging traditional medical knowledge with modern communication channels. A Chiropractic Physician with specialized certifications, Dr. Curtis has carved out a unique space in healthcare education that goes far beyond conventional boundaries.

While his professional journey spans talk radio, academic lecture halls, newspaper columns, and public speaking, Dr. Curtis has recently found a dynamic new platform on TikTok. With nearly half a million followers, he has emerged as a digital health sage, delivering clear, natural, and accessible health advice that cuts through medical jargon and speaks directly to people's everyday wellness concerns.

His newsletter, Long Life Healthy Life, and his upcoming podcast have become a thriving community of health-conscious individuals seeking comprehensive, actionable wellness insights. Through this platform, Dr. Curtis continues to expand his reach, offering in-depth articles, personal health strategies, and a supportive network for those committed to long-term well-being.

Dr. Curtis approaches health with a refreshing practicality, offering guidance that feels more like advice from a trusted friend than a distant medical professional. His commitment to demystifying health challenges and presenting natural solutions has made him a beacon for those seeking authentic, straightforward wellness information.

Whether addressing complex health questions or exploring holistic approaches to well-being, Dr. Curtis continues to be a trusted navigator in the complex landscape of personal health, helping individuals understand and take control of their wellness journey.

www.ingramcontent.com/pod-product-compliance
Lightning Source LLC
Chambersburg PA
CBHW061047250726
48653CB00001B/290